The Complete Guide to Full-Body Stretching

Improve Mobility, Reduce Pain, and Enhance Your Wellbeing

Helen Talbott

Copyright © [2024] [Helen Talbott]

All rights reserved.

This book is protected by copyright. No part of this book may be reproduced or transmitted in any form or by any means, electronic or mechanical, including photocopying, recording, or by any information storage and retrieval system, without written permission from the author.

Disclaimer

The information contained in this book is for informational purposes only and is not intended as a substitute for professional medical advice, diagnosis, or treatment. Always consult with a qualified healthcare professional before starting any new exercise program, especially if you have any injuries or medical conditions.

The author and publisher disclaim any liability for any injury or health problems that may arise from the use of the information contained in this book.

Table of content

About the author

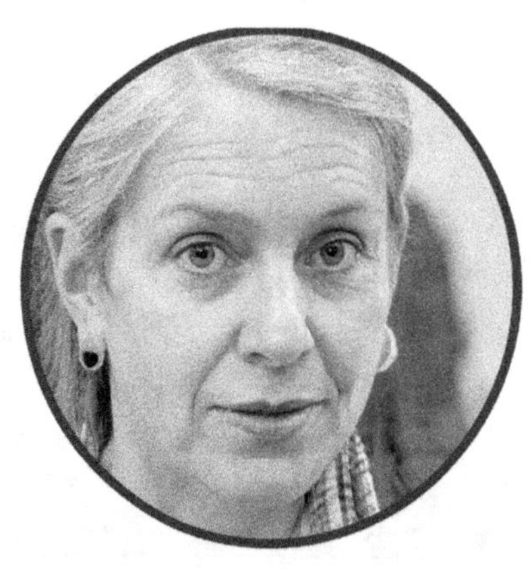

Helen Talbott is a passionate advocate for health and well-being through movement and mindful practices. Her own journey of incorporating stretching into her life to improve flexibility and manage occasional aches and pains sparked a desire to share the benefits with others.

Drawing on her extensive research and experience in fitness and wellness, Helen crafts accessible and informative resources to empower individuals to take charge of their mobility and live a vibrant, active life. She believes that stretching is not just about physical benefits, but also a gateway to relaxation, stress reduction, and a deeper connection with your body.

Beyond the Book:

Helen is a regular contributor to health and fitness publications, offering practical stretching routines and tips for beginners and experienced exercisers alike. She also conducts workshops and online courses, making stretching knowledge accessible to a wider audience.

When Helen isn't immersed in the world of stretching, you might find her exploring nature, practicing yoga, or whipping up healthy and delicious meals in her kitchen. Her passion for a holistic approach to wellness shines through in everything she does.

Introduction

The Secret Language Your Body Speaks (and How to Listen with Stretches)

Imagine your body as a magnificent temple, housing your spirit and potential. But over time, dust settles in the corners, cobwebs drape the rafters, and the doors creak in protest. This, my friend, is what happens when we neglect our flexibility.

The good news? Your body whispers a secret language, a symphony of aches, stiffness, and limited movement. By learning to stretch, we become fluent in this language, translating those whispers into powerful commands for increased mobility, reduced pain, and a newfound sense of freedom.

This book isn't just about touching your toes (although, hey, that's a bonus!). It's about unlocking the hidden potential within you. It's about becoming a master negotiator with your muscles, coaxing them into releasing tension and rediscovering their natural range of motion.

Within these pages, we'll embark on a journey of discovery, deciphering the language of your body. We'll explore different stretching techniques, crafting personalized routines that address your unique needs. Whether you're an athlete yearning for peak performance, a weekend warrior just starting out, or simply someone seeking a pain-free life, you'll find the tools and knowledge to transform your relationship with your body.

So, silence the creaks, banish the cobwebs, and prepare to unleash your inner flexibility. Let the stretching begin!

Chapter 1

Unleash Your Inner Flexibility (or Why Stretch?)

Ever feel like a rusty hinge? You reach for that coffee mug on the top shelf, and your shoulder lets out a groan of protest. Or maybe you dream of gracefully bending over to touch your toes, but your hamstrings feel like iron cables. These are all signs that your inner flexibility is yearning to be unleashed.

But why stretch? It's more than just a pre-workout routine or a fancy yoga pose. Stretching is like a magic key that unlocks a treasure trove of benefits for your body and mind. Here's why you should become a master of this powerful tool:

- **Effortless Movement, Like a Well-Oiled Machine:** Imagine bending down to pick up a dropped pen without a wince, or performing daily tasks with the ease of a dancer. Stretching lengthens your muscles, allowing you to move with fluidity and confidence, making even the most mundane activities a joy.

- **Become Injury-Proof:** Tight muscles are like ticking time bombs, waiting to explode into a painful strain or tear. Stretching increases blood flow, keeping your muscles loose and prepared for action. This significantly reduces your risk of injuries, especially during exercise.

- **Kiss Bad Posture Goodbye:** Poor posture can lead to a domino effect of aches, pains, and even long-term health problems. Stretching targets the muscles that contribute to bad posture, promoting better alignment and a more confident appearance. You'll stand taller, feel stronger, and radiate confidence from the inside out.

- **Stress Less, Live More:** Stretching isn't just about the physical; it's a powerful mind-body connection. Holding a gentle stretch allows your body to relax and unwind, promoting stress reduction and a sense of calm. It's the perfect antidote to the daily grind, leaving you feeling centered and ready to take on the world.

This Book is for Everyone:

The beauty of stretching lies in its universality. Whether you're a seasoned athlete pushing your limits, a weekend warrior just starting out, or someone leading a more sedentary life, incorporating stretching into your routine can make a world of difference.

- **Athletes:** Stretching is the secret weapon for peak performance. Increased flexibility allows for greater athletic range of motion, leading to better technique, efficiency, and potentially even improved results.
- **Beginners:** Stretching helps prepare your body for new activities and reduces the risk of injury as you embark on your fitness journey.
- **People with Pain:** Stretching can help alleviate pain caused by tight muscles and

improve mobility in people with conditions like arthritis or back pain.

No matter your age, fitness level, or specific goals, this chapter is your invitation to unlock the power of stretching and transform your approach to health, well-being, and movement. So, take a deep breath, let's begin!

Why this book

This book, *The Complete Guide to Full-Body Stretching: Improve Mobility, Reduce Pain, and Enhance Your Wellbeing*, is your one-stop shop for unlocking the hidden potential within you through stretching. Here's why this book is the perfect companion on your journey to a more flexible and pain-free you:

- **Unveils the Power of Stretching:** Forget the misconception of stretching as just a pre-workout chore. This book dives deep into the numerous benefits, from improved mobility and reduced pain to stress relief and better posture.
- **Crafts Personalized Routines:** It goes beyond generic stretches. You'll learn about different techniques and how to tailor a program to your specific needs and goals, whether you're an athlete or someone seeking pain relief.
- **Focuses on Safety and Accessibility:** Whether you're a beginner or have existing injuries, this book emphasizes

proper form, modifications, and when to listen to your body.

- **Offers a Roadmap for Long-Term Success:** It's not just about the quick fix. This book equips you with the knowledge and tools to integrate stretching into your daily routine for lasting results.
- **Clear and Engaging Writing:** The book uses clear and engaging language, making complex topics easy to understand and implement.

In short, this book is more than just a collection of stretches. It's your guide to becoming fluent in the language of your body, unlocking a world of benefits, and taking control of your health and well-being.

The Importance of Flexibility in Modern Life: More Than Just Touching Your Toes

In our fast-paced, desk-bound world, flexibility often takes a backseat. But the truth is, cultivating flexibility is more important than ever in modern life. It's not just about achieving the perfect yoga pose or finally touching your toes (although those are great achievements!). Here's why flexibility is a key ingredient for a healthy and fulfilling life:

Enhanced Mobility and Daily Function:

Think about your daily routine. Bending down to pick up groceries, reaching for that high shelf, or even tying your shoes – all these seemingly simple tasks require a certain degree of flexibility. Tight muscles can make these movements cumbersome and even painful. Stretching regularly increases your range of motion, allowing you to move with ease and confidence in your everyday activities.

Reduced Risk of Injury:

Tight muscles are like wound-up springs, prone to snapping. Stretching increases blood flow to your muscles, keeping them loose and prepared for movement. This significantly reduces your risk of injuries, especially during exercise or sudden movements. Athletes swear by stretching for a reason – it helps them perform at their peak while minimizing the risk of getting sidelined.

Improved Posture and Body Awareness:

Poor posture can lead to a domino effect of aches, pains, and even long-term health problems. Stretching targets the muscles that contribute to bad posture, promoting better alignment and a more confident appearance. Additionally, stretching improves body awareness, helping you understand your limitations and avoid awkward positions or movements that could lead to injury.

Stress Relief and Relaxation:

The mind and body are deeply connected. Holding a gentle stretch allows your body to relax and unwind, promoting stress reduction and a sense of calm. Stretching can be a form of active meditation, helping you release tension and find inner peace.

Lifelong Benefits for Overall Well-being:

The benefits of flexibility extend far beyond the physical. As we age, maintaining flexibility becomes even more crucial. It helps us stay mobile and independent, reducing the risk of falls and injuries. Stretching can also improve our balance and coordination, allowing us to navigate the world with greater confidence.

Making Flexibility a Modern Necessity:

Modern life often traps us in a cycle of inactivity. Long hours spent sitting at desks contribute to muscle tightness and a decline in flexibility. Stretching offers a powerful antidote. By incorporating it into your daily routine, even for just a few minutes, you can counteract the negative effects of a sedentary lifestyle and unlock the numerous benefits of a flexible body.

So, ditch the misconception of stretching as just a pre-workout routine. Embrace it as a vital tool for a healthy, active, and fulfilling life in our modern world.

The Transformative Power of Stretching: Unveiling a Multitude of Benefits

In our fast-paced world, prioritizing physical activity often takes center stage. While cardio and strength training are crucial for overall health, stretching deserves equal recognition. It's not just about the ability to touch your toes or achieve a picture-perfect yoga pose; stretching offers a treasure trove of benefits that extend far beyond increased flexibility. Here's a deep dive into the transformative power of stretching and how it can significantly enhance your life:

Enhanced Mobility and Functional Movement:

Imagine navigating your daily routine with ease and confidence. Stretching lengthens your muscles, increasing your range of motion. This translates to simple tasks like bending down to pick up groceries, reaching for high shelves, or tying your shoes becoming a breeze. Tight muscles can make these movements cumbersome and even painful. Stretching regularly ensures you move with fluidity and efficiency, eliminating unnecessary strain on your body.

Reduced Risk of Injury:

Think of your muscles as elastic bands. When tight and unused, they're more prone to snapping. Stretching increases blood flow to your muscles, keeping them loose and prepared for action. This significantly reduces your risk of injuries, especially during exercise or sudden movements. Athletes swear by stretching for a reason – it helps them push their limits while minimizing the risk of getting sidelined.

Improved Posture and Body Awareness:

Poor posture can wreak havoc on your body, leading to aches, pains, and even long-term health problems. Stretching targets the muscles that contribute to bad posture, promoting better alignment. This translates to a more confident appearance and improved balance. Additionally, stretching enhances body awareness. You become more attuned to your limitations and can avoid awkward positions or movements that could lead to injury.

Stress Relief and Relaxation:

The mind and body are intricately connected. Holding a gentle stretch allows your body to relax and unwind, promoting stress reduction and a sense of calm. Stretching can be a form of active meditation, helping you release tension and find inner peace. In today's world, chronic stress is a major concern. Stretching provides a powerful antidote, allowing you to de-stress and find a sense of centeredness.

Enhanced Athletic Performance:

For athletes, stretching is a non-negotiable element of their training routine. Increased flexibility translates to greater athletic range of motion, leading to better technique, efficiency, and potentially improved results. Whether you're a runner, a weightlifter, or a team sport athlete, stretching helps you perform at your peak by ensuring proper form and reducing the risk of injury.

Improved Circulation and Blood Flow:

Stretching increases blood flow to your muscles, delivering essential nutrients and oxygen. This not only improves muscle function but also helps remove waste products like lactic acid, which can contribute to fatigue and soreness. Improved circulation can also benefit your overall cardiovascular health by lowering blood pressure and reducing the risk of heart disease.

Pain Management and Injury Recovery:

Tight muscles can contribute to chronic pain conditions like back pain and muscle tension. Stretching helps alleviate pain by lengthening and loosening tight muscles, improving blood flow, and reducing inflammation. Additionally, stretching plays a crucial role in injury recovery by promoting healing and restoring proper range of motion.

Enhanced Sleep Quality:

Struggling to get a good night's sleep? Stretching can be the answer. By promoting relaxation and reducing stress, stretching prepares your body for restful sleep. It also helps release muscle tension that can keep you awake at night. So, incorporate a gentle stretching routine before bed and experience the difference on your sleep quality.

Lifelong Benefits for Overall Well-being:

The benefits of flexibility extend far beyond the physical. As we age, maintaining flexibility becomes even more crucial. It helps us stay mobile and independent, reducing the risk of falls and injuries. Stretching can also improve our balance and coordination, allowing us to navigate the world with greater confidence.

A Gateway to Mindfulness and Body Connection:

Stretching can be a meditative practice, encouraging you to focus on your breath and become more aware of your body's sensations.

This mindful approach fosters a deeper connection with your body, allowing you to appreciate its capabilities and limitations.

In Conclusion:

Stretching is an often-overlooked yet vital component of a healthy lifestyle. It's a practice that offers a multitude of benefits, from improved mobility and reduced pain to stress relief and enhanced athletic performance. Regardless of your age, fitness level, or specific goals, incorporating stretching into your routine is an investment in your overall well-being. So, take a deep breath, reach for the sky, and unlock the transformative power of stretching!

This is just a starting point, and you can tailor the content to the specific focus of your book. You can add details on different stretching techniques or create sections focused on the benefits for specific populations (e.g., athletes, beginners, older adults).

Stretching: A Universal Language for Everyone

The beauty of stretching lies in its universality. It's a practice that transcends age, fitness level, or specific goals. Whether you're a seasoned athlete pushing your limits, a weekend warrior just starting your journey, or someone leading a more sedentary life, incorporating stretching into your routine can make a world of difference. Here's how stretching benefits diverse groups:

Athletes:

For athletes, stretching is a non-negotiable element of their training. Increased flexibility allows for greater athletic range of motion, leading to:

- **Improved Technique:** Proper form is crucial for peak performance and injury prevention. Stretching helps athletes achieve deeper positions, execute movements with better control, and maximize their efficiency.

- **Enhanced Performance:** Greater flexibility allows athletes to move with greater fluidity and power, potentially leading to improved results in their chosen sport.
- **Reduced Risk of Injury:** Tight muscles are more susceptible to strains and tears. Stretching keeps muscles loose and prepared for intense activity, minimizing the risk of injuries that can sideline athletes.

Weekend Warriors and Fitness Beginners:

Starting a new exercise routine can be daunting, and the fear of injury is a common concern. Stretching plays a crucial role in preparing your body for new activities:

- **Injury Prevention:** Just like with athletes, stretching helps reduce the risk of injury by keeping muscles loose and prepared for the demands of unfamiliar movements.

- **Improved Range of Motion:** As you embark on your fitness journey, stretching helps you gradually increase your range of motion, allowing you to perform exercises with better form and efficiency.
- **Enhanced Enjoyment:** When your body feels loose and limber, you're more likely to enjoy your workouts and stay motivated to continue your fitness journey.

People with Pain or Injuries:

Living with pain or recovering from an injury can be frustrating. Stretching offers a gentle yet effective way to manage pain and promote healing:

- **Pain Relief:** Tight muscles can contribute to chronic pain conditions like back pain and muscle tension. Stretching helps alleviate pain by lengthening and loosening tight muscles, improving blood flow, and reducing inflammation.
- **Improved Mobility:** Stretching helps restore proper range of motion after an

injury, aiding in the healing process and promoting a faster return to normal activities.

- **Pain Management:** Stretching can be a valuable tool for pain management, helping individuals manage chronic pain conditions and improve their overall quality of life.

People with Sedentary Lifestyles:

Those who lead desk jobs or have limited physical activity can reap significant benefits from stretching:

- **Improved Posture:** Sitting for long periods can contribute to poor posture. Stretching targets the muscles that contribute to bad posture, promoting better alignment and potentially reducing aches and pains.
- **Increased Mobility:** A sedentary lifestyle can lead to muscle stiffness and a decline in flexibility. Regular stretching helps counteract these effects, improving your

range of motion and making daily
activities easier.

- **Stress Relief:** Stretching can be a form of
active meditation, promoting relaxation
and reducing stress levels. This can be
particularly beneficial for those who
experience chronic stress due to their
work or lifestyle.

Older Adults:

Maintaining flexibility is crucial as we age.
Stretching offers numerous benefits for older
adults:

- **Improved Balance and Coordination:**
Stretching helps improve balance and
coordination, reducing the risk of falls and
injuries, which are a major concern for
older adults.

- **Enhanced Mobility:** Maintaining
flexibility allows older adults to stay
mobile and independent for longer,
performing daily tasks with greater ease
and confidence.

- **Pain Management:** Stretching can help alleviate pain caused by arthritis and other age-related conditions, improving overall well-being and quality of life.

In Conclusion:

Stretching is a gift you can give your body at any age or stage of life. Regardless of your background or goals, incorporating stretching into your routine is an investment in your health and well-being. So, take a deep breath, embrace the benefits, and embark on your journey to a more flexible and fulfilling you!

Chapter 2

Mastering the Art of Stretching - Understanding Different Techniques

Just like learning a new language, mastering the art of stretching requires understanding different techniques. Each technique offers unique benefits and is best suited for specific situations. Here, we'll delve into the three main categories of stretching techniques:

1. Static Stretching:

This is the most common type of stretching, often associated with yoga or cool-down routines. It involves holding a gentle stretch for a sustained period, typically 15-30 seconds.

- **Benefits:**
    - Increases flexibility by lengthening shortened muscles.
    - Improves range of motion.

- o Promotes relaxation and stress relief.
- **When to Use:**
  - o As part of a cool-down routine after exercise.
  - o To improve overall flexibility.
  - o To maintain flexibility gains made through other stretching techniques.

2. Dynamic Stretching:

Dynamic stretching involves controlled movements that gradually prepare your muscles for activity. It's a fantastic way to warm up your body before exercise.

- **Benefits:**
  - o Increases blood flow and prepares muscles for movement.
  - o Improves coordination and agility.
  - o Reduces the risk of injury during exercise.
- **When to Use:**
  - o As part of a warm-up routine before exercise.

    ○ To improve athletic performance.

    ○ To activate and prepare muscles for specific movements.

Examples of Dynamic Stretches:

- Leg Swings (forward and backward)

- Arm Circles (forward and backward)

- Walking Lunges with Torso Twists

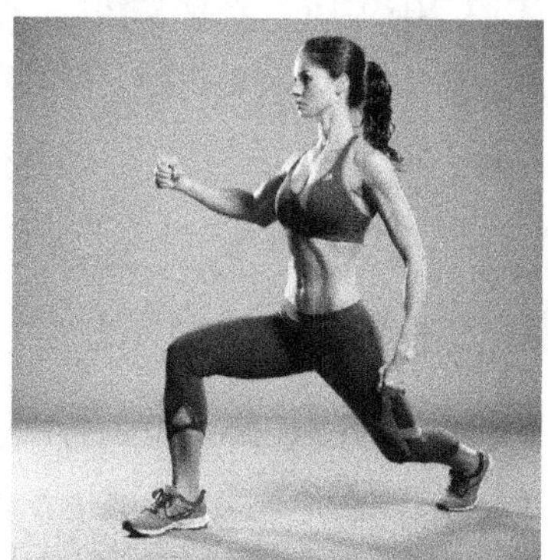

- High Knees

3. PNF (Proprioceptive Neuromuscular Facilitation) Stretching:

PNF stretching is a more advanced technique that involves a combination of isometric contractions (muscle tensing) and assisted stretches. It's best practiced under the guidance of a qualified professional.

- **Benefits:**
    - May lead to deeper flexibility gains compared to static stretching alone.
    - Can be helpful for targeting specific muscle imbalances.
- **When to Use:**
    - Under the supervision of a qualified professional (e.g., physical therapist, athletic trainer).
    - For athletes seeking to maximize their flexibility gains.
    - For individuals with specific muscle imbalances or tightness.

Important Considerations:

- **Always listen to your body.** Stretching should cause a slight pulling sensation, not pain. If you feel pain, stop the stretch and consult a healthcare professional.

- **Proper breathing is key.** Inhale slowly and deeply as you enter the stretch, and exhale slowly as you hold it.
- **Maintain good form.** Don't bounce or jerk during stretches. Aim for smooth, controlled movements.
- **Be consistent.** Regular stretching is crucial for maintaining and improving flexibility. Aim for at least a few minutes of stretching most days of the week.

Choosing the Right Technique:

The best stretching technique depends on your specific goals and situation. Here's a quick guide:

- **For a cool-down or overall flexibility improvement:** Static stretching is a great choice.
- **For a warm-up or to improve athletic performance:** Dynamic stretching is ideal.

- **For deeper flexibility gains or addressing muscle imbalances (under guidance):** Consider PNF stretching.

By understanding these different techniques and their applications, you can create a personalized stretching routine that unlocks your full potential and helps you achieve your flexibility goals.

Mastering Proper Stretching Form: The Key to Safe and Effective Flexibility Gains

Stretching is a powerful tool for unlocking a world of benefits, but reaping those rewards hinges on proper form. Just like any physical activity, improper technique can lead to injury and hinder your progress. This section delves into the essential elements of good stretching form, ensuring you embark on a safe and effective journey towards greater flexibility.

The Foundation: Alignment and Posture

- **Neutral Spine:** Imagine your spine as a stack of blocks. Maintain a neutral position throughout most stretches, avoiding excessive rounding of the back or arching of the lower back.
- **Engaged Core:** A strong core provides stability and protects your lower back. Engage your core muscles by drawing your navel slightly inwards as you enter the stretch.

- **Hip Alignment:** Keep your hips square and avoid rolling them inwards or outwards during stretches. This ensures proper alignment and prevents unnecessary strain on your hips and knees.

Movement and Breath: The Dynamic Duo

- **Controlled Movements:** Stretching should be a gradual and controlled process. Avoid bouncing or jerking, as this can lead to muscle tears. Move smoothly and mindfully into each stretch.
- **Slow and Deep Breaths:** Breathing plays a crucial role in stretching. Inhale slowly and deeply through your nose as you enter the stretch, allowing your body to relax. Exhale slowly through your mouth as you hold the stretch. Focus on your breath and use it to manage any discomfort.

Finding Your Edge: Intensity and Duration

- **Listen to Your Body:** Stretching should never be painful. Aim for a gentle pulling sensation, indicating that you're targeting the right muscles. If you feel pain, stop the stretch and consult a healthcare professional.

- **Hold for the Right Time:** For static stretches, aim to hold each position for 15-30 seconds. This allows your muscles sufficient time to lengthen and relax.
- **Gradual Progression:** Don't push yourself too hard, especially when starting. Gradually increase the intensity and duration of your stretches as your flexibility improves.

Additional Tips for Optimal Form:

- **Warm Up Before Stretching:** Always perform a light warm-up before stretching, especially static stretching. This increases blood flow and prepares your muscles for movement.
- **Focus on Isolation:** Target specific muscle groups with each stretch. Isolate the muscle you're trying to stretch and

avoid engaging other muscle groups unnecessarily.

- **Don't Hold Your Breath:** Holding your breath during stretches can strain your heart and reduce the effectiveness of the stretch. Breathe continuously and deeply throughout the entire process.
- **Maintain Proper Alignment Throughout:** Pay attention to your form throughout the entire stretch, not just at the beginning. Ensure your body remains aligned and avoid compromising your posture.

Remember: Consistency is Key

Stretching is not a one-time event; it's an ongoing practice. Aim to incorporate short stretching sessions (5-10 minutes) into your daily routine, or at least several times a week. Consistency is crucial for maintaining and improving your flexibility.

By following these guidelines and focusing on proper stretching form, you can maximize the benefits of your stretches and minimize the risk of injury. As you progress, you'll develop a keen awareness of your body and its limitations, allowing you to refine your technique and personalize your stretching routine for optimal results. Happy stretching!

When to Stretch: Optimizing Your Routine for Maximum Benefit

Stretching is a powerful tool, but timing it right can significantly enhance its effectiveness. Here's a breakdown of the ideal times to incorporate stretching into your routine:

Warm-up Stretches (Dynamic):

- **Before Exercise:** This is a non-negotiable! Perform dynamic stretches 5-10 minutes before any physical activity.
- **Benefits:**
  - Increases blood flow and prepares muscles for movement.
  - Improves range of motion and reduces the risk of injury during exercise.
  - Enhances coordination and agility.
- **Examples:** Leg Swings, Arm Circles, Walking Lunges with Torso Twists, High Knees.

Cool-down Stretches (Static):

- **After Exercise:** Stretch for 10-15 minutes after your workout when your muscles are warm and pliable.
- **Benefits:**
    - Lengthens muscles and improves flexibility.
    - Reduces muscle soreness and stiffness.
    - Promotes relaxation and aids in recovery.
- **Examples:** Hamstring Stretch, Quad Stretch, Calf Stretch, Chest Stretch, Shoulder Stretches.

Additional Stretching Opportunities:

- **Throughout the Day:** Short stretching breaks (5-10 minutes) can be beneficial, especially for those who sit for long periods.
- **Before Bed:** Gentle static stretches can help relax your muscles and prepare you for a restful night's sleep.

- **Active Recovery Days:** Stretching on rest days helps maintain flexibility and promotes recovery from previous workouts.

Listen to Your Body:

While these are general guidelines, the best time to stretch is whenever your body feels tight or stiff. Pay attention to your body's signals, and incorporate stretching as needed throughout the day.

Here's a quick summary table:

Type of Stretch	When to Do It	Benefits
Dynamic Stretches	Before Exercise (5-10 minutes)	Increases blood flow, improves range of motion, reduces injury risk

Static Stretches	After Exercise (10-15 minutes)	Improves flexibility, reduces soreness, promotes relaxation
Short Stretches	Throughout the Day (5-10 minutes)	Improves mobility, reduces stiffness
Gentle Stretches	Before Bed	Promotes relaxation, improves sleep quality
Stretches	Active Recovery Days	Maintains flexibility, aids recovery

Remember: Consistency is key! Aim to incorporate stretching into your routine regularly, even if it's just for a few minutes a day. By strategically incorporating stretches throughout your day, you'll maximize the benefits and unlock your full potential for flexibility and improved well-being.

https://docs.google.com/spreadsheets/d/1sAJbmnek8A36wzIsn10Gp6hVC0FsYjmN3P1aVaOlR7M/edit?usp=drivesdk

Here's the link to a quick summary table

Chapter 3

Building Your Personalized Stretching Routine

Crafting Your Personalized Stretching Journey: A Guide to Tailoring a Program for Your Needs

The beauty of stretching lies in its versatility. Unlike a one-size-fits-all approach, stretching can be customized to address your unique needs and goals. Whether you're a seasoned athlete, a weekend warrior just starting out, or someone seeking pain relief, this chapter empowers you to create a personalized stretching program that unlocks your inner flexibility and enhances your overall well-being.

Step 1: Identify Your Goals and Needs

The foundation of your personalized stretching program begins with a clear understanding of your goals and needs. Here are some key questions to consider:

- **What is your current level of flexibility?** Are you a beginner with limited mobility, or do you have a foundation of flexibility you want to build upon?
- **What is your fitness level?** Are you an athlete seeking peak performance, or are you leading a more sedentary lifestyle and aiming to improve overall mobility?
- **Do you have any specific injuries or limitations?** Certain stretches may need to be modified or avoided depending on any existing injuries or pain points.
- **What are your overall fitness goals?** Are you training for a specific event, seeking to improve your posture, or simply looking to reduce stress and improve your quality of life?

By reflecting on these questions, you gain a clearer picture of where you are currently and where you want to be with your flexibility.

Step 2: Choose Your Stretches:

With your goals in mind, explore the different stretching techniques covered in Chapter 2 (Static, Dynamic, PNF). Here's a roadmap to guide your selection:

- **For Overall Flexibility Improvement:** Static stretches are a great choice. Focus on major muscle groups like hamstrings, quads, calves, chest, back, shoulders, and neck.
- **For Improved Athletic Performance:** Dynamic stretches are ideal for a pre-workout warm-up. Choose stretches that target the specific muscles used in your chosen sport or activity.
- **For Pain Relief and Injury Recovery:** Consult a qualified professional (physical therapist, athletic trainer) to design a program that addresses your specific needs. They can recommend modified stretches to target tight areas and promote healing.

Step 3: Tailor and Modify:

No two bodies are alike. What works for one person might not be suitable for another. Here's how to personalize your routine:

- **Focus on Tight Areas:** Pay attention to areas that feel particularly tight or stiff. Dedicate more time to stretches that target these specific muscle groups.
- **Modify for Limitations:** If you have any injuries or limitations, research modifications for common stretches. Alternatively, consult a healthcare professional who can design a safe and effective program based on your individual needs.
- **Listen to Your Body:** Pain is never your friend. If you feel any sharp pain during a stretch, stop immediately and consult a healthcare professional. Stretching should never be uncomfortable; aim for a gentle pulling sensation.

Step 4: Structure Your Routine:

Now that you have your stretches chosen and any necessary modifications made, it's time to structure your routine:

- **Warm-up (Before Exercise):** Perform dynamic stretches for 5-10 minutes before any physical activity.
- **Cool-down (After Exercise):** Dedicate 10-15 minutes to static stretches after your workout when your muscles are warm and pliable.
- **Throughout the Day:** Aim for short stretching breaks (5-10 minutes) throughout the day, especially if you sit for long periods.
- **Active Recovery Days:** Don't neglect stretching on rest days! Light stretching helps maintain flexibility and promotes recovery from previous workouts.

Step 5: Consistency is Key:

The magic of stretching lies in consistent practice. Aim to incorporate stretching into your routine regularly, even if it's just for a few minutes a day. Over time, you'll experience a gradual increase in flexibility, improved range of motion, and a reduction in muscle soreness and stiffness.

Additional Tips:

- **Create a Stretching Sanctuary:** Dedicate a quiet space in your home where you can comfortably stretch. Use calming music or aromatherapy to create a relaxing atmosphere.
- **Set Realistic Goals:** Don't expect to become a contortionist overnight. Set realistic and achievable goals to stay motivated on your stretching journey.
- **Track Your Progress:** Use a journal or app to track your progress. This can help you stay motivated and celebrate your achievements.
- **Enjoy the Process:** Focus on the feeling of relaxation and rejuvenation that stretching brings to your body and mind. Embrace the journey and enjoy the benefits of a more flexible you!

Stretching Essentials: Equipping Yourself for a Successful Flexibility Journey

While stretching requires minimal equipment, having a few key items can enhance your comfort, safety, and overall experience. Here's a breakdown of the various tools you might consider incorporating into your stretching routine:

The Fundamentals: Comfort and Support

- **Stretching Mat:** This is the foundation of your stretching sanctuary. Invest in a comfortable, non-slip mat that provides cushioning and support for your body. Look for mats with a thickness of 1/4 inch to 1/2 inch, offering a balance between comfort and stability.
- **Yoga Strap:** A yoga strap can be a valuable tool to deepen stretches and target specific muscle groups. Straps can be used to assist with poses that require greater flexibility or to improve your form. Look for straps made from durable

yet comfortable materials like cotton or nylon.

- **Yoga Blocks:** Yoga blocks provide additional support and stability during stretches. They can help you achieve proper alignment and allow you to hold stretches more comfortably. Blocks come in various materials like cork, foam, or wood. Choose blocks that are firm yet comfortable and the right size for your needs.

Enhancing Your Practice: Tools for Deeper Stretches

- **Foam Roller:** This self-massage tool helps release muscle tension and improve circulation. Foam rolling can be particularly beneficial before stretching as it helps prepare your muscles for deeper stretches. Choose a foam roller with varying densities depending on your preference and sensitivity.
- **Massage Balls:** Similar to foam rollers, massage balls can be used to target

specific trigger points and tight areas. They're ideal for pinpoint pressure and releasing tension in smaller muscle groups like the feet and hands. Choose massage balls with different textures depending on your desired level of intensity.

- **Stretch Bands:** Resistance bands can add a dynamic element to your stretching routine. They can be used for assisted stretches or to create gentle resistance, promoting strength and flexibility simultaneously. Choose bands with varying levels of resistance to accommodate your current fitness level.

Considerations and Safety Tips:

- **Quality Matters:** Invest in good quality equipment that is durable and comfortable to use. Look for materials that are free of harmful chemicals and are easy to clean.
- **Start Simple:** You don't need a lot of equipment to get started. Begin with a basic mat and explore your stretching

practice before investing in additional tools.

- **Listen to Your Body:** Never use any equipment that causes pain or discomfort. If unsure about using a specific tool, consult a healthcare professional or qualified instructor.
- **Focus on Proper Form:** Equipment is meant to enhance your stretching, not replace proper form. Ensure you maintain good alignment and listen to your body's signals during each stretch.

Beyond the Essentials: Creating Your Stretching Sanctuary

- **Comfortable Clothing:** Wear loose-fitting, comfortable clothing that allows for freedom of movement during your stretches. Opt for breathable fabrics like cotton or moisture-wicking materials to stay comfortable throughout your practice.
- **Calming Music:** Set the mood for relaxation with calming music or nature

sounds. Create a playlist that promotes a sense of peace and tranquility during your stretching routine.

- **Aromatherapy:** Essential oils like lavender or chamomile can be used to create a relaxing atmosphere. Diffuse essential oils or use scented candles (with caution) to enhance your stretching experience.

Remember: Consistency is key! Regardless of the equipment you choose, the most important element is dedication to your stretching routine. With regular practice and the right tools, you'll be well on your way to achieving greater flexibility and a more fulfilling journey towards a healthier and more mobile you.

Chapter 4

Conquering Neck and Shoulder Tightness

Taming the Tightness: Effective Stretches for Upper Traps, Neck Flexors, and Rotator Cuff Muscles

The upper body, particularly the neck, shoulders, and upper back, are notorious for harboring tension. Tightness in the upper traps, neck flexors, and rotator cuff muscles can lead to pain, headaches, and limitations in movement. This section dives deep into effective stretches to target these specific muscle groups, promoting relaxation, improved posture, and a pain-free upper body.

Understanding the Muscles:

- **Upper Traps:** The upper trapezius muscles run along the upper back and neck, connecting the shoulder blades to the spine. Tight upper traps can contribute to neck pain, headaches, and poor posture.

- **Neck Flexors:** The neck flexor muscles are located at the front of the neck and are responsible for bending your head forward. Overuse of these muscles from prolonged computer work or looking down at phones can lead to neck pain and stiffness.

- **Rotator Cuff Muscles:** The rotator cuff muscles are a group of four muscles that surround the shoulder joint, providing stability and allowing for a wide range of motion. Tightness or weakness in these muscles can lead to shoulder pain and impingement.

Stretching Strategies:

1. Upper Traps:

- **Chin Tucks:** Sit or stand tall with good posture. Gently tuck your chin down towards your chest, lengthening the back of your neck and engaging your upper back muscles. Hold for 15-30 seconds and repeat 3-5 times.

- **Neck Rolls:** Slowly roll your head in a circular motion, leading with your chin and keeping your shoulders relaxed. Complete 5-10 rolls in each direction.
- **Doorway Chest Opener:** Stand in a doorway with your forearms on either side of the doorframe. Gently lean forward, feeling a stretch across your chest and upper back. Hold for 15-30 seconds and repeat 3-5 times.

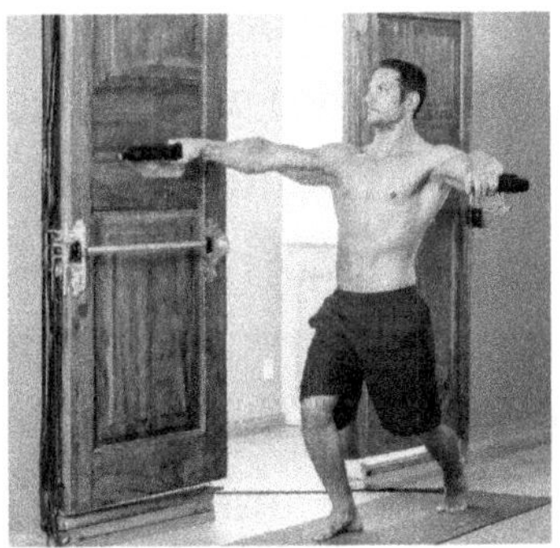

2. Neck Flexors:

- **Neck Retractions:** Sit or stand tall with good posture. Gently push your head back as if creating a "double chin" without straining. Hold for 15-30 seconds and repeat 3-5 times. This stretch targets the deep neck flexors.

- **Foam Rolling:** Lie on your back with a foam roller placed horizontally across your upper back. Slowly roll your head back and forth across the foam roller, applying gentle pressure to target tight spots in your upper neck muscles. Avoid placing direct pressure on your spine.
- **Supine Neck Stretch:** Lie on your back with your knees bent and feet flat on the floor. Slowly turn your head to one side, keeping your shoulders relaxed. Use your hand on the opposite side of your head to provide gentle pressure, increasing the stretch without straining. Hold for 15-30 seconds per side and repeat 3-5 times.

3. Rotator Cuff Muscles:

- **Arm Circles:** Stand tall with your arms outstretched to the sides at shoulder height. Make small, controlled circles forward for 10 repetitions, then reverse directions and perform 10 circles backward. Keep your shoulders relaxed and focus on initiating the movement from your shoulder blades.

- **Doorway Shoulder Stretch:** Stand in a doorway with one arm raised overhead and your forearm against the doorframe. Lean gently into the doorway, feeling a stretch in the front of your shoulder. Hold for 15-30 seconds and repeat 3-5 times per side.
- **Cross-body Arm Stretch:** Stand tall with your arms extended out to the sides at shoulder height. Gently pull your left arm across your body with your right hand, stretching the back of your left shoulder. Hold for 15-30 seconds and repeat 3-5 times per side.

Important Tips:

- **Breathe:** Inhale slowly and deeply as you enter the stretch, and exhale slowly as you hold it. Focus on your breath and use it to manage any discomfort.

- **Listen to Your Body:** Pain is never a good sign. If you feel any sharp pain during a stretch, stop immediately and consult a healthcare professional. Stretching should feel like a gentle pulling sensation.
- **Hold and Repeat:** Hold each stretch for 15-30 seconds and repeat 3-5 times for each exercise.
- **Consistency is Key:** Incorporate these stretches into your daily routine, even if it's just for a few minutes a day. Regular stretching is crucial for maintaining and improving flexibility.

Additional Considerations:

- **Strengthening Exercises:** Stretching is just one piece of the puzzle. Strengthening the muscles around your upper back, neck, and shoulders can help improve posture and prevent future tightness. Consider exercises like rows

Combating Headaches and Cultivating Posture: Effective Stretches for a Pain-Free You

Tension headaches and poor posture are two common woes that can plague people of all ages. The good news is that these issues are often intertwined, and a targeted stretching routine can be a powerful weapon in your arsenal for combating both. This section delves into effective stretches that address these concerns, promoting a pain-free and well-aligned posture.

Understanding the Connection:

- **Tightness and Posture:** Poor posture, often characterized by rounded shoulders and a hunched upper back, can lead to tightness in the chest, neck, and upper back muscles. This tightness can pull your head out of alignment, contributing to tension headaches.
- **The Domino Effect:** Conversely, headaches can also lead to poor posture. The discomfort of a headache can cause

you to subconsciously tense your neck and shoulder muscles, further perpetuating the cycle of pain.

Stretching Strategies:

Here are some key stretches to target the muscle groups most commonly associated with tension headaches and poor posture:

1. Upper Traps and Neck:

- **Chin Tucks:** Sit or stand tall with good posture. Gently tuck your chin down towards your chest, lengthening the back of your neck and engaging your upper back muscles. Hold for 15-30 seconds and repeat 3-5 times.
- **Neck Rolls:** Slowly roll your head in a circular motion, leading with your chin and keeping your shoulders relaxed. Complcte 5-10 rolls in each direction.
- **Neck Retractions:** Sit or stand tall with good posture. Gently push your head back as if creating a "double chin" without

straining. Hold for 15-30 seconds and repeat 3-5 times. This stretch targets the deep neck flexors.

2. Chest and Shoulders:

- **Doorway Chest Opener:** Stand in a doorway with your forearms on either side of the doorframe. Gently lean forward, feeling a stretch across your chest and upper back. Hold for 15-30 seconds and repeat 3-5 times.
- **Arm Circles:** Stand tall with your arms outstretched to the sides at shoulder height. Make small, controlled circles forward for 10 repetitions, then reverse directions and perform 10 circles backward. Keep your shoulders relaxed and focus on initiating the movement from your shoulder blades.
- **Cross-body Arm Stretch:** Stand tall with your arms extended out to the sides at shoulder height. Gently pull your left arm across your body with your right hand, stretching the back of your left shoulder.

Hold for 15-30 seconds and repeat 3-5 times per side.

3. Additional Stretches for Improved Posture:

- **Foam Rolling Upper Back:** Lie on your back with a foam roller placed horizontally across your upper back. Slowly roll your back and forth across the foam roller, applying gentle pressure to target tight spots. Avoid placing direct pressure on your spine.
- **Child's Pose:** Kneel on the floor with your toes together and knees hip-width apart. Sit back on your heels and rest your forehead on the floor, stretching your arms out in front of you. Hold for 30 seconds to 1 minute.
- **Cat-Cow Stretch:** Start on your hands and knees with your wrists under your shoulders and hips under your knees. Inhale as you arch your back and lift your head and tailbone (cow pose). Exhale as you round your back, tucking your chin to

your chest (cat pose). Repeat for several cycles.

Enhancing the Effects:

- **Strengthening Exercises:** Stretching is just one piece of the puzzle. Strengthening your core and upper back muscles can help improve posture and prevent future tightness. Consider exercises like rows, planks, and supermans.
- **Ergonomics:** Pay attention to your posture throughout the day, especially when sitting at a desk. Ensure your chair provides proper back support and adjust your workstation to maintain good alignment.
- **Mind-Body Connection:** Techniques like mindfulness meditation can help you become more aware of your posture and tension patterns. By focusing on your breath and relaxing your body, you can further combat tension headaches.

Remember: Consistency is Key!

Incorporate these stretches into your daily routine, even if it's just for a few minutes a day. Over time, you'll experience a reduction in tension headaches, improved flexibility in your neck and shoulders, and a more aligned and pain-free posture.

By combining these stretches with a focus on ergonomics and posture awareness, you can break the cycle of tension and discomfort, paving the way for a healthier and more pain-free you!

Chapter 5

Unlocking Back Flexibility and Pain Relief

Releasing Tension and Finding Freedom: Stretches for a Mobile Thoracic Spine, Lumbar Spine, and Core

The spine, our body's central support system, comprises three key regions: the cervical spine (neck), the thoracic spine (upper back), and the lumbar spine (lower back). Alongside these regions lies the core, a network of muscles that provide stability and power for movement. Tightness or stiffness in any of these areas can lead to pain, limited mobility, and difficulty performing everyday tasks. This section dives deep into effective stretches for the thoracic spine, lumbar spine, and core muscles, promoting a more mobile and pain-free spine.

Understanding the Importance of Mobility:

- **Thoracic Spine:** The thoracic spine, located in the upper back, has a natural curve that allows for rotation and extension. Tightness in this area can restrict breathing, contribute to poor posture, and lead to pain between the shoulder blades.
- **Lumbar Spine:** The lumbar spine, located in the lower back, has a natural inward curve that supports the weight of the upper body. Tightness in this area can lead to lower back pain, disc issues, and limited flexibility.
- **Core Muscles:** The core muscles, including the abdominals, obliques, and lower back muscles, provide stability and power for movement. Weak or tight core muscles can contribute to back pain, poor posture, and difficulty maintaining balance.

Stretching Strategies:

Here are some key stretches to target each of these crucial areas:

1. Thoracic Spine:

- **Foam Rolling Upper Back:** Lie on your back with a foam roller placed horizontally across your upper back. Slowly roll your back and forth across the foam roller, applying gentle pressure to target tight spots. Avoid placing direct pressure on your spine.
- **Doorway Chest Opener:** Stand in a doorway with your forearms on either side of the doorframe. Gently lean forward, feeling a stretch across your chest and upper back. Hold for 15-30 seconds and repeat 3-5 times.
- **Thoracic Spine Rotations:** Sit or stand tall with your arms outstretched to the sides at shoulder height. Gently rotate your torso to one side, keeping your hips facing forward. Hold for 15-30 seconds and repeat on the other side. Complete 3-5 repetitions per side.

2. Lumbar Spine:

- **Cat-Cow Stretch:** Start on your hands and knees with your wrists under your shoulders and hips under your knees. Inhale as you arch your back and lift your head and tailbone (cow pose). Exhale as you round your back, tucking your chin to your chest (cat pose). Repeat for several cycles.
- **Knee to Chest Stretches:** Lie on your back with both knees bent and feet flat on the floor. Hug one knee to your chest, holding for 15-30 seconds. Gently lower your knee and repeat with the other leg. Perform 3-5 repetitions per side.
- **Supine Twist:** Lie on your back with both knees bent and feet flat on the floor. Gently lower both knees to one side, keeping your shoulders grounded and looking in the opposite direction. Hold for 15-30 seconds and repeat on the other side. Perform 3-5 repetitions per side.

3. Core Muscles:

- **Bird-Dog:** Start on your hands and knees with your wrists under your shoulders and hips under your knees. Extend one arm and the opposite leg out straight, keeping your back flat and core engaged. Hold for 15-30 seconds and repeat on the other side. Perform 3-5 repetitions per side.

- **Plank:** Start in a push-up position with your forearms on the floor. Keep your body in a straight line from head to heels, engaging your core muscles. Hold for 30 seconds to 1 minute, gradually increasing the hold time as you get stronger.

- **Dead Bug:** Lie on your back with your knees bent and feet flat on the floor. Extend one arm straight up towards the ceiling and the opposite leg straight out, keeping your lower back pressed into the floor. Slowly lower your arm and leg back down without letting your back arch. Repeat on the other side. Perform 3-5 repetitions per side.

Important Considerations:

- **Breathe:** Inhale slowly and deeply as you enter the stretch, and exhale slowly as you hold it. Focus on your breath and use it to manage any discomfort.
- **Listen to Your Body:** Pain is never a good sign. If you feel any sharp pain during a stretch, stop immediately and consult a healthcare professional. Stretching should feel like a gentle pulling sensation.
- **Hold and Repeat:** Hold each stretch for 15-30 seconds and repeat 3-5 times for each exercise.

Chapter 6

Opening Up Your Chest and Arms

Unleash Your Inner Archer: Effective Stretches for Chest Tightness and Enhanced Shoulder Mobility

Tightness in the chest and limited shoulder mobility can be a real drag, hindering everyday activities and athletic performance. Whether you're a weekend warrior or simply someone who spends a lot of time hunched over a desk, this section equips you with effective stretches to target these areas, promoting a more open chest, improved posture, and a wider range of motion in your shoulders.

Understanding the Culprits:

- **Chest Tightness:** Tightness in the chest muscles, particularly the pectoralis major and minor, can arise from various factors like prolonged sitting, poor posture, and certain activities like weightlifting. This tightness can restrict your breathing, limit shoulder mobility, and contribute to rounded shoulders.

- **Limited Shoulder Mobility:** The shoulder joint is a ball-and-socket joint, allowing for a wide range of motion. However, tightness in the surrounding muscles like the rotator cuff and deltoids can restrict this range of motion, leading to pain and difficulty performing overhead movements.

Stretching Strategies:

Here are some key stretches to address both chest tightness and limited shoulder mobility:

1. Chest Stretches:

- **Doorway Chest Opener:** This classic stretch is a grcat way to open up the chest muscles. Stand in a doorway with your forearms on either side of the doorframe. Gently lean forward, feeling a stretch across your chest and upper back. Hold for 15-30 seconds and repeat 3-5 times.

- **Foam Rolling Pectorals:** Lie on a foam roller with a tennis ball placed underneath each armpit. Slowly roll back and forth across the foam roller, applying gentle pressure to target tight spots in your chest muscles. Avoid placing direct pressure on your ribs or bones.
- **Arm Circles:** Stand tall with your arms outstretched to the sides at shoulder height. Make small, controlled circles forward for 10 repetitions, then reverse directions and perform 10 circles backward. Keep your shoulders relaxed and focus on initiating the movement from your shoulder blades.

2. Shoulder Mobility Stretches:

- **Arm Circles with Reach:** Stand tall and extend your arms overhead. Make small, controlled circles with your arms, gradually increasing the size of the circles as you feel comfortable. Perform 10 circles forward and 10 circles backward.

- **Cross-body Arm Stretch:** Stand tall with your arms extended out to the sides at shoulder height. Gently pull your left arm across your body with your right hand, stretching the back of your left shoulder. Hold for 15-30 seconds and repeat 3-5 times per side.

- **Sleeper Stretch:** Lie on your stomach with your head turned towards one side and your top arm extended overhead. Gently press your palm into the floor or a yoga block to create a gentle stretch in the front of your shoulder. Hold for 15-30 seconds and repeat on the other side.

Enhancing Your Routine:

- **Dynamic Stretches:** Before any physical activity, incorporate dynamic stretches like arm circles, arm swings, and shoulder rolls to warm up your shoulder joint and prepare it for movement.

- **Strengthening Exercises:** Complement your stretching routine with exercises that strengthen the muscles around your shoulders. This helps improve stability and prevent future tightness. Consider exercises like rows, overhead presses, and external rotations.
- **Proper Posture:** Maintaining good posture throughout the day, especially when sitting, helps prevent tightness in the chest and shoulders. Focus on keeping your shoulders back and down, and avoid slouching.

Important Considerations:

- **Breathe:** Inhale slowly and deeply as you enter the stretch, and exhale slowly as you hold it. Focus on your breath and use it to manage any discomfort.
- **Listen to Your Body:** Pain is never a good sign. If you feel any sharp pain during a stretch, stop immediately and consult a healthcare professional.

Stretching should feel like a gentle pulling sensation.

- **Consistency is Key:** Incorporate these stretches into your daily routine, even if it's just for a few minutes a day. Over time, you'll experience a more open chest, improved shoulder mobility, and a wider range of motion in your upper body.

Bonus Tip: Consider incorporating yoga or Pilates into your exercise routine. These practices often include stretches and exercises that specifically target the chest, shoulders, and upper back, promoting overall mobility and flexibility.

By following these strategies and remaining consistent, you'll be well on your way to unlocking a more mobile and pain-free upper body. Remember, proper form and listening to your body are crucial for achieving optimal results. Happy stretching!

Stretches for Enhanced Reach and Reduced Injury Risk: Expanding Your Range of Motion Safely

Reaching for that top shelf or that perfect overhead smash in tennis – good flexibility goes a long way in daily life and athletic performance. But flexibility training isn't just about showing off your range of motion; it's a crucial component of injury prevention. Here, we explore targeted stretches to increase your reach and keep you moving pain-free.

Understanding Flexibility and Injury Prevention:

- **Importance of Reach:** Increased reach allows for greater efficiency in daily activities and improved performance in various sports. From grabbing objects to swinging a golf club, good flexibility helps you move with ease and power.
- **Injury Prevention:** Tight muscles are more prone to tears and strains. Stretching helps improve the elasticity of your

muscles, allowing them to absorb force and prevent injuries during sudden movements.

Stretching Strategies for Increased Reach:

Here are some key stretches to target the major muscle groups that contribute to reach:

- **Upper Body:**
  - **Doorway Chest Opener:** A classic! Stand in a doorway with your forearms on either side of the frame. Lean forward, feeling a stretch across your chest and shoulders. Hold for 15-30 seconds and repeat 3-5 times.
  - **Arm Circles:** Stand tall with arms outstretched to the sides. Make small, controlled circles forward and backward (10 repetitions each direction). Keep shoulders relaxed and initiate the movement from your shoulder blades.

- **Lat Pulldown Stretch with Towel (or Band):** Sit on the floor with legs extended. Loop a towel (or resistance band) under your feet and hold the ends overhead. Gently lean back, feeling a stretch in your lats and upper back. Hold for 15-30 seconds and repeat 3-5 times.
- **Core and Lower Body:**
  - **Hamstring Stretch:** Sit on the floor with one leg extended and the other bent with your foot flat on the floor. Lean forward, reaching towards your toes, keeping your back straight. Hold for 15-30 seconds and repeat on the other side (3-5 repetitions per leg).
  - **Quad Stretch:** Stand on one leg and grab the ankle of your other leg behind you. Gently pull your heel towards your glutes, feeling a stretch in the front of your thigh. Hold for 15-30 seconds and repeat

on the other side (3-5 repetitions per leg).

- ○ **Spinal Twist:** Sit on the floor with your knees bent and feet flat. Rotate your torso to one side, keeping your hips facing forward and looking over your shoulder. Hold for 15-30 seconds and repeat on the other side (3-5 repetitions per side).

Maximizing Your Stretches for Injury Prevention:

- **Dynamic Stretches:** Before any physical activity, incorporate dynamic stretches like arm swings, leg swings, and torso twists to warm up your muscles and prepare them for movement.
- **Hold and Repeat:** Aim to hold each static stretch for 15-30 seconds and repeat 3-5 times. Consistency is key!
- **Listen to Your Body:** Pain is never a good sign. If you feel any sharp pain during a stretch, stop immediately.

Breathe deeply and focus on a gentle pulling sensation.

- **Strengthening Exercises:** Complement your stretching with exercises that target the stretched muscles. This helps improve stability and prevent future tightness. Consider exercises like rows, lunges, and planks.
- **Proper Form:** Maintain good posture throughout your stretches. Avoid bouncing or forcing the stretch.

Bonus Tip: Consider incorporating yoga or Pilates into your routine. These practices often include stretches and exercises that specifically target the muscles for reach and injury prevention, promoting overall flexibility and core strength.

Remember: Consistency is key! By incorporating these stretches into your daily routine and maintaining proper form, you'll be well on your way to achieving greater reach, improved performance, and a reduced risk of injuries. Happy stretching!

Chapter 7

Enhancing Hip and Leg Flexibility

Conquering the Lower Body: Effective Stretches for Hamstrings, Quads, Hip Flexors, and Calves

The lower body is a powerhouse, propelling us through daily activities and athletic endeavors. However, tight muscles in the hamstrings, quads, hip flexors, and calves can lead to pain, limited mobility, and decreased performance. This section delves into effective stretches for each of these crucial muscle groups, ensuring a limber lower body and a foundation for pain-free movement.

Understanding the Importance of Flexibility:

- **Improved Mobility:** Tightness in any of these lower body muscle groups can restrict your range of motion, making activities like squatting, lunging, and running feel awkward and inefficient. Stretching improves flexibility, allowing for smoother and more efficient movement.

- **Reduced Pain and Injury Risk:** Tight muscles are more prone to strains and tears. Stretching helps increase the elasticity of your muscles, allowing them to absorb force and prevent injuries during sudden movements.
- **Enhanced Performance:** Improved flexibility in the lower body translates to better athletic performance. From deeper squats to more powerful strides, increased flexibility allows you to move with greater ease and power.

Stretching Strategies:

1. Hamstrings:

- **Standing Forward Fold:** Stand tall with your feet hip-width apart. Hinge at your hips and fold forward, reaching towards your toes (or shins if you can't reach your toes comfortably). Keep a slight bend in your knees and your back flat. Hold for 15-30 seconds and repeat 3-5 times.

- **Lying Hamstring Stretch:** Lie on your back with one leg extended and the other bent with your foot flat on the floor. Loop a yoga strap or towel around the arch of your extended foot and gently pull it towards you, feeling a stretch in the back of your thigh. Hold for 15-30 seconds and repeat on the other side (3-5 repetitions per leg).

2. Quads:

- **Standing Quad Stretch:** Stand on one leg and grab the ankle of your other leg behind you. Gently pull your heel towards your glutes, feeling a stretch in the front of your thigh. Hold for 15-30 seconds and repeat on the other side (3-5 repetitions per leg).
- **Quad Stretch with Support:** Lie on your stomach with one leg bent and your foot

flat on the floor. Reach back and grab your ankle or foot (if comfortable). Gently pull your heel towards your glutes, feeling a stretch in the front of your thigh. If you can't reach your foot, loop a towel or yoga strap around your ankle and use it to assist the stretch. Hold for 15-30 seconds and repeat on the other side (3-5 repetitions per leg).

3. Hip Flexors:

- **Kneeling Hip Flexor Stretch:** Start in a kneeling position with one knee on the floor and the other leg extended in front of you. Lean your hips forward, keeping your back straight, until you feel a stretch in the front of your hip on the kneeling leg. Hold for 15-30 seconds and repeat on the other side (3-5 repetitions per leg).
- **Pigeon Pose:** Start on your hands and knees and bring one knee forward, placing it between your hands. Slide your other leg back, keeping your hips square. Lean your torso forward, keeping your back

straight, until you feel a stretch in the front of your hip on the extended leg. Hold for 15-30 seconds and repeat on the other side (3-5 repetitions per leg).

4. Calves:

- **Downward-Facing Dog Calf Stretch:** Start in a downward-facing dog position (hands and feet hip-width apart) with your heels pressing towards the floor. Walk your heels back towards your hands, keeping your legs straight, until you feel a stretch in your calves. Hold for 15-30 seconds and repeat 3-5 times.
- **Wall Calf Stretch:** Stand facing a wall with your hands shoulder-width apart on the wall. Step one leg back, keeping your heel flat on the floor. Lean into the wall, keeping your front leg straight, until you feel a stretch in your calf. Hold for 15-30 seconds and repeat on the other side (3-5 repetitions per leg).

Maximizing Your Stretches:

- **Dynamic Stretches:** Before any physical activity, incorporate dynamic stretches like leg swings, lunges with twists, and high knees to warm up your lower body muscles and prepare them for movement.
- **Hold and Repeat:** Aim to hold each static stretch for 15-30 seconds and repeat 3-5 times. Consistency is key!
- **Listen to Your Body:** Pain is never a good sign. If you feel any sharp pain during a stretch, stop immediately. Breathe deeply and focus

Unleashing Your Inner Athlete: Stretches for Enhanced Range of Motion and Injury Prevention

A body in motion stays in motion, but a body with limited range of motion can lead to pain, frustration, and increased risk of injury. Stretching is a fundamental tool for athletes and non-athletes alike, promoting greater flexibility, improved performance, and a reduced risk of getting sidelined. This section dives deep into effective stretches for various muscle groups, helping you unlock a wider range of motion and move with confidence.

The Power of Flexibility:

- **Enhanced Range of Motion (ROM):** Flexibility allows your joints to move through a greater range of motion. This translates to smoother and more efficient movement in everyday activities like reaching for objects, bending down, or climbing stairs.

- **Injury Prevention:** Tight muscles are more susceptible to strains and tears. Stretching helps increase the elasticity of your muscles, allowing them to absorb force and adapt to sudden movements, thus reducing the risk of injuries.
- **Improved Performance:** Greater flexibility in key muscle groups can enhance athletic performance. From deeper squats for weightlifters to a more powerful kick for soccer players, flexibility allows for better mechanics and potentially improved results.

Stretching Strategies for Increased ROM:

Here are some key stretches to target major muscle groups and improve overall range of motion:

Upper Body:

- **Chest:**
    - **Doorway Chest Opener:** A classic! Stand in a doorway with

your forearms on either side of the doorframe. Lean forward, feeling a stretch across your chest and shoulders. Hold for 15-30 seconds and repeat 3-5 times.

- **Arm Circles:** Stand tall with arms outstretched to the sides at shoulder height. Make small, controlled circles forward and backward (10 repetitions each direction). Keep shoulders relaxed and focus on initiating the movement from your shoulder blades.

- **Shoulders:**
  - **Cross-body Arm Stretch:** Stand tall with your arms extended out to the sides at shoulder height. Gently pull your left arm across your body with your right hand, stretching the back of your left shoulder. Hold for 15-30 seconds and repeat 3-5 times per side.
  - **Sleeper Stretch:** Lie on your stomach with your head turned

towards one side and your top arm extended overhead. Gently press your palm into the floor or a yoga block to create a gentle stretch in the front of your shoulder. Hold for 15-30 seconds and repeat on the other side.

- **Back:**
    - **Cat-Cow Stretch:** Start on your hands and knees with your wrists under your shoulders and hips under your knees. Inhale as you arch your back and lift your head and tailbone (cow pose). Exhale as you round your back, tucking your chin to your chest (cat pose). Repeat for several cycles.
    - **Foam Rolling Upper Back:** Lie on a foam roller with your upper back placed on it. Slowly roll back and forth, applying gentle pressure to target tight spots in your upper back muscles. Avoid placing direct pressure on your spine.

Lower Body:

- **Hamstrings:**
  - **Standing Forward Fold:** Stand tall with your feet hip-width apart. Hinge at your hips and fold forward, reaching towards your toes (or shins if you can't reach your toes comfortably). Keep a slight bend in your knees and your back flat. Hold for 15-30 seconds and repeat 3-5 times.
  - **Lying Hamstring Stretch:** Lie on your back with one leg extended and the other bent with your foot flat on the floor. Loop a yoga strap or towel around the arch of your extended foot and gently pull it towards you, feeling a stretch in the back of your thigh. Hold for 15-30 seconds and repeat on the other side (3-5 repetitions per leg).
- **Quads:**

- ○ **Standing Quad Stretch:** Stand on one leg and grab the ankle of your other leg behind you. Gently pull your heel towards your glutes, feeling a stretch in the front of your thigh. Hold for 15-30 seconds and repeat on the other side (3-5 repetitions per leg).
  - ○ **Quad Stretch with Support:** Lie on your stomach with one leg bent and your foot flat on the floor. Reach back and grab your ankle or foot (if comfortable). Gently pull your heel towards your glutes, feeling a stretch in the front of your thigh. If you can't reach your foot, loop a towel or yoga strap around your ankle and use it to assist the stretch. Hold for 15-30 seconds and repeat on the other side (3-5 repetitions per leg).
- **Calves:**
  - ○ **Downward-Facing Dog Calf Stretch:** Start in a

downward-facing   dog   position
(hands and feet hip-width apart)
with your heels pressing towards

Chapter 8

Crafting the Perfect Stretch Routine

Ignite Your Workout: Dynamic Stretches for a Pre-Workout Warm-up

A dynamic warm-up is an essential first step to any effective workout. It prepares your body for movement by gently increasing your heart rate, blood flow, and muscle temperature. Unlike static stretches (holding a position for a sustained period), dynamic stretches involve controlled movements that mimic the actions you'll be performing during your workout. This section delves into effective dynamic stretches to prime your body for peak performance and reduce your risk of injury.

The Benefits of Dynamic Stretches:

- **Enhanced Performance:** Dynamic stretches activate your nervous system and prepare your muscles for the demands of your workout, potentially leading to improved coordination, power, and agility.

- **Reduced Injury Risk:** By increasing blood flow and muscle temperature, dynamic stretches can help loosen tight muscles and improve range of motion, making your body more resilient to strains and tears.
- **Mental Preparation:** A dynamic warm-up can help you mentally focus and transition smoothly into your workout routine.

Dynamic Stretches for a Powerful Warm-up:

Here are some key dynamic stretches to target major muscle groups and prepare your body for various types of workouts:

Full Body:

- **Arm Circles:** Stand tall with your arms outstretched to the sides at shoulder height. Make small, controlled circles forward and backward for 10 repetitions each direction. Keep your shoulders relaxed and focus on initiating the movement from your shoulder blades.

Lower Body:

- **Leg Swings:** Stand on one leg and swing the other leg forward and backward in a controlled manner, keeping your core engaged. Repeat for 10-15 swings per leg.
- **High Knees:** Run in place while bringing your knees up high towards your chest. Focus on maintaining good form and keeping your core tight. Perform for 30-60 seconds.
- **Butt Kicks:** Run in place while kicking your heels up towards your glutes. Maintain good posture and keep your core engaged. Perform for 30-60 seconds.
- **Lunges with Twists:** Step forward into a lunge, then twist your torso towards the front leg as you reach your arms overhead. Repeat on the other side. Perform 10 lunges with twists per leg.

Upper Body:

- **Arm Swings:** Stand tall with your arms by your sides. Swing your arms back and forth in a controlled manner, gradually increasing the range of motion as you feel comfortable. Perform for 30 seconds.
- **Shoulder Rolls:** Roll your shoulders forward in a circular motion for 10 repetitions, then reverse directions and roll them backward for 10 repetitions.

Core:

- **Walking Plank:** Start in a high plank position with your hands shoulder-width apart and your body in a straight line from head to heels. Step one foot out to the side, then bring it back to the starting position and repeat with the other leg. Continue this "walking" motion for 30-60 seconds.
- **Russian Twists:** Sit on the floor with your knees bent and feet flat on the ground. Lean back slightly, keeping your core

engaged, and twist your torso from side to side, reaching your arms towards the ground on each side. Perform 10-15 twists per side.

Remember:

- **Perform each dynamic stretch for 30-60 seconds or 10-15 repetitions.**
- **Focus on controlled movements and proper form.**
- **Breathe deeply and rhythmically throughout the warm-up.**
- **Tailor your dynamic stretches to your specific workout routine.**

By incorporating these dynamic stretches into your pre-workout routine, you'll be well on your way to a safe and successful workout. Remember, a proper warm-up is an investment in your performance and injury prevention. So, get moving, loosen up, and unleash your inner athlete!

Soothing Your Muscles: Effective Static Stretches for a Post-Workout Cool-down

After a challenging workout, your body craves a proper cool-down. This allows your heart rate and blood pressure to return to normal, helps flush out metabolic waste products, and promotes muscle recovery. Static stretches, which involve holding a position for a sustained period (15-30 seconds), are a crucial part of the cool-down routine. Here, we explore effective static stretches to target major muscle groups, promoting flexibility, reducing muscle soreness, and aiding in post-workout recovery.

The Importance of Post-Workout Stretching:

- **Improved Flexibility:** Stretching after a workout, when your muscles are warm and pliable, can help improve your overall flexibility over time. This can lead to better range of motion and potentially enhance your athletic performance.
- **Reduced Muscle Soreness:** Static stretches can help reduce post-workout

muscle soreness, also known as Delayed Onset Muscle Soreness (DOMS). By gently lengthening tight muscles, you can minimize discomfort and promote faster recovery.

- **Enhanced Blood Flow:** Holding static stretches can help improve blood flow to your muscles, which can further aid in the removal of metabolic waste products produced during exercise.

Static Stretches for a Complete Cool-down:

Here are some key static stretches to target major muscle groups commonly worked during various workouts:

Upper Body:

- **Chest:**
    - **Doorway Chest Opener:** A classic cool-down stretch! Stand in a doorway with your forearms on either side of the doorframe. Lean forward, feeling a stretch across

your chest and shoulders. Hold for 15-30 seconds and repeat 3-5 times.

- **Arm Circles (Slow and Controlled):** Stand tall with your arms outstretched to the sides at shoulder height. Make slow, controlled circles forward and backward for 10 repetitions each direction.

- **Shoulders and Back:**
  - **Cross-body Arm Stretch:** Stand tall with your arms extended out to the sides at shoulder height. Gently pull your left arm across your body with your right hand, stretching the back of your left shoulder. Hold for 15-30 seconds and repeat 3-5 times per side.
  - **Cat-Cow Stretch (Modified):** Start on your hands and knees with your wrists under your shoulders and hips under your knees. Inhale as you arch your back and lift your head and chest slightly (modified

cow pose). Exhale as you round your back and tuck your chin to your chest (cat pose). Repeat for several cycles.

Lower Body:

- **Hamstrings:**
  - **Standing Forward Fold:** Stand tall with your feet hip-width apart. Hinge at your hips and fold forward, reaching towards your toes (or shins if you can't reach your toes comfortably). Keep a slight bend in your knees and your back flat. Hold for 15-30 seconds and repeat 3-5 times.
- **Quads:**
  - **Quad Stretch with Support:** Lie on your stomach with one leg bent and your foot flat on the floor. Reach back and grab your ankle or foot (if comfortable). Gently pull your heel towards your glutes, feeling a stretch in the front of your

thigh. If you can't reach your foot, loop a towel or yoga strap around your ankle and use it to assist the stretch. Hold for 15-30 seconds and repeat on the other side (3-5 repetitions per leg).

- **Calves:**
  - **Downward-Facing Dog Calf Stretch:** Start in a downward-facing dog position (hands and feet hip-width apart) with your heels pressing towards the floor. Walk your heels back towards your hands, keeping your legs straight, until you feel a stretch in your calves. Hold for 15-30 seconds and repeat 3-5 times.

Additional Tips for a Complete Cool-down:

- **Light Cardio:** Incorporate 5-10 minutes of light cardio, such as walking or jogging, after your static stretches. This helps your heart rate gradually return to normal.

- **Deep Breathing:** Focus on deep, diaphragmatic breathing throughout your cool-down routine. This helps promote relaxation and recovery.
- **Hydration:** Don't forget to rehydrate after your workout. Drinking plenty of water helps replenish fluids lost through sweat and aids in muscle recovery.

By incorporating these static stretches into your post-workout cool-down routine, you'll be giving your body the TLC it needs to recover effectively and bounce back stronger for your next workout. Remember, consistency is key! The more you stretch, the more flexible you'll become, and the less likely you are to experience muscle soreness. So stretch, breathe, and recover like a champ!

Unwind and Recharge: Stretches for Relaxation and Improved Sleep

The modern world can leave us feeling wired and restless, making it difficult to drift off to sleep at night. Stretching, often overlooked as a relaxation technique, can be a powerful tool for promoting calmness, reducing tension, and preparing your body for restful sleep. This section explores gentle stretches that target major muscle groups, helping you ease into a relaxed state and improve your overall sleep quality.

The Power of Stretching for Sleep:

- **Reduced Muscle Tension:** Throughout the day, muscles accumulate tension, especially in areas like the neck, shoulders, and lower back. Stretching these areas helps release tension, promoting a sense of physical relaxation that can carry over into your sleep.
- **Improved Blood Flow:** Gentle stretches can improve blood flow throughout the

body, promoting relaxation and helping your body wind down. This improved circulation may also aid in the removal of metabolic waste products that can contribute to feelings of restlessness.

- **Mind-Body Connection:** The act of stretching encourages a focus on your breath and your body's sensations. This mindfulness can help quiet a racing mind and promote a sense of calm, preparing you for sleep.

Stretching Strategies for a Restful Night:

Here are some key stretches to target major muscle groups and promote relaxation before bed:

Upper Body:

- **Neck Stretches:**
    - **Gentle Side Bends:** Sit or stand tall with good posture. Slowly tilt your head to one side, bringing your ear towards your shoulder. Hold for

15-30 seconds and repeat on the other side (2-3 repetitions per side).

- ○ **Chin Tucks:** Sit or stand tall with good posture. Gently tuck your chin down towards your chest, lengthening the back of your neck. Hold for 15-30 seconds and repeat 2-3 times.

- **Shoulder Stretches:**
  - ○ **Arm Circles (Slow and Controlled):** Stand tall with your arms outstretched to the sides at shoulder height. Make slow, controlled circles forward and backward for 10 repetitions each direction. Focus on keeping your shoulders relaxed and initiating the movement from your shoulder blades.
  - ○ **Doorway Chest Opener (Modified):** Stand in a doorway with your forearms on either side of the frame at a lower level (approximately chest height).

Gently lean forward, feeling a mild stretch across your chest and shoulders. Hold for 15-30 seconds and repeat 2-3 times.

Lower Body:

- **Hamstring Stretch (Supine):** Lie on your back with both legs extended. Loop a yoga strap or towel around the arch of one foot and gently pull it towards you, feeling a stretch in the back of your thigh. Hold for 15-30 seconds and repeat on the other side (2-3 repetitions per leg).
- **Quad Stretch (Modified):** Lie on your stomach with one leg bent and your foot flat on the floor. Gently squeeze your glutes of the bent leg. Hold for 15-30 seconds and repeat on the other side (2-3 repetitions per leg).

Additional Tips for a Relaxing Stretches Routine:

- **Create a Calming Environment:** Dim the lights, put on calming music, or light some aromatherapy candles to create a relaxing atmosphere for your stretches.

- **Focus on Your Breath:** Incorporate deep, diaphragmatic breathing throughout your stretches. Inhale slowly through your nose and exhale slowly through your mouth. Focus on the sensation of your breath entering and leaving your body.

- **Listen to Your Body:** These stretches should feel gentle and relaxing. If you feel any pain, stop the stretch immediately.

- **Hold for Shorter Durations:** Unlike stretches for flexibility, hold these stretches for 15-30 seconds each, focusing on gentle tension rather than pushing your limits.

- **Make it a Routine:** Incorporate these stretches into your bedtime routine 30-60 minutes before sleep for optimal benefits.

Complementary Practices for Better Sleep:

- **Warm Bath:** Taking a warm bath before bed can help raise your body temperature and then allow it to drop slightly afterward, mimicking the natural sleep cycle and promoting relaxation.
- **Relaxation Techniques:** Practices like progressive muscle relaxation or meditation can further enhance the calming effects of stretching and promote better sleep.
- **Limiting Screen Time:** The blue light emitted from electronic devices can disrupt sleep patterns. Avoid screens for at least an hour before bedtime.

By incorporating these gentle stretches and relaxation techniques into your routine, you can create a powerful sleep ritual that helps you unwind, reduce tension, and drift off to a more restful sleep. Remember, consistency is key! The more you prioritize relaxation practices before bed, the better your sleep quality will become. Sweet dreams!

Chapter 9

Making Stretching a Habit You Love

Weaving Stretches Seamlessly into Your Day: Practical Tips for Consistent Stretching

Stretching is a well-known yet often underutilized tool for maintaining flexibility, improving mobility, and enhancing overall well-being. However, incorporating it into your daily routine can feel like a challenge. Here are some practical tips to help you seamlessly integrate stretching into your day, making it a sustainable habit:

Pair Stretching with Existing Activities:

- **Morning Stretch Ritual:** Wake up your body and mind with gentle stretches before you even get out of bed. Reach for your toes, roll your shoulders, and stretch your side body.
- **Post-Workout Cool Down:** Dedicate 5-10 minutes after your workout to stretches that target major muscle groups used during your activity.

- **Pre-Bed Routine:** Wind down for a restful sleep with some relaxing stretches that focus on your back, hamstrings, and shoulders.
- **Commercial Breaks:** During commercial breaks while watching TV, get up and perform some standing stretches like leg swings, arm circles, or calf raises.

Make Stretching Convenient and Accessible:

- **Keep Stretches Short and Simple:** Aim for 15-30 second holds for each stretch, focusing on proper form rather than duration. Short and effective stretches are easier to incorporate into your busy schedule.
- **Utilize Technology:** Download a stretching app that provides guided routines or set reminders on your phone to prompt yourself for stretching breaks.
- **Turn it into a Family Activity:** Make stretching a fun family activity! Stretch together after dinner or turn it into a playful game, encouraging each other and keeping things light.
- **Stretch While You Wait:** Waiting in line at the grocery store or for your coffee? Use that time for some simple calf raises, ankle circles, or neck stretches.

Focus on Consistency Over Perfection:

- **Small Wins Matter:** Don't get discouraged if you can't stretch every single day. Even a few minutes of stretching a few times a week can make a difference.
- **Listen to Your Body:** Pay attention to your body's signals. If you feel pain, stop the stretch. Stretching should never be uncomfortable.
- **Find Stretches You Enjoy:** Experiment with different stretches and find ones you find enjoyable. This will increase your motivation to stick with it.
- **Track Your Progress:** Use a journal or app to track your progress. Noting improvements in flexibility or reduced pain can be a great motivator.

Remember: Consistency is key! By incorporating these tips, you can transform stretching from a chore to a natural part of your daily routine, paving the way for a more flexible, mobile, and vibrant you. So, get stretching, and experience the multitude of benefits it has to offer!

Conquering Common Stretching Obstacles: Motivation and Time Crunches

We all know the benefits of stretching: improved flexibility, reduced pain, and a more limber body. Yet, incorporating stretching into our daily lives can be a struggle. Let's tackle two common roadblocks – motivation and time constraints – and explore strategies to overcome them:

Motivation Meltdown:

- **Identify Your "Why":** Remind yourself why stretching is important to you. Do you want to improve your athletic performance? Reduce back pain? Enhance your overall well-being? A clear purpose can reignite your motivation.
- **Set Realistic Goals:** Don't aim to become a contortionist overnight. Start with small, achievable goals, like stretching for 5 minutes after work three times a week. Celebrating small victories will keep you motivated.
- **Find a Stretching Buddy:** Having a friend or family member to stretch with can add a layer of fun and accountability. Partner up and motivate each other!

- **Visualize Success:** Imagine how you'll feel after a good stretch – more relaxed, less achy, and ready to move with ease. Visualization can be a powerful tool for boosting motivation.
- **Reward Yourself:** Celebrate your commitment to stretching! After a consistent week, treat yourself to a relaxing bath or a healthy smoothie. Positive reinforcement keeps you on track.

Time Tightrope Walk:

- **Short Bursts, Big Benefits:** You don't need a dedicated hour to reap the benefits of stretching. Even short bursts throughout the day can make a difference.
- **Stretch While You Wait:** Waiting in line or for your coffee to brew? Utilize those brief moments for calf raises, ankle circles, or neck stretches. Every little bit counts!
- **Multitask Your Stretches:** Combine stretching with other activities. Watch TV while doing seated stretches, listen to music while stretching your legs before bed, or hold a light stretch while talking on the phone.
- **Stretch During Your Commute:** If you take public transportation, use that time for some

gentle stretches. Focus on your neck, shoulders, and legs.

- **Incorporate Micro-Stretches:** Make stretching a mindful practice throughout your day. Roll your shoulders while sitting at your desk, stretch your calves while brushing your teeth, or reach for your toes while picking something up off the floor.

Remember: Consistency is key! Even short, regular stretching sessions are far more beneficial than occasional long ones. Embrace these strategies, find what works for you, and transform stretching into a manageable and rewarding habit. Start small, stay consistent, and witness the positive impact stretching can have on your life!

Chapter 10

Exploring Advanced Stretching Techniques

Deep Dive into PNF Stretching: Unlocking Advanced Flexibility

For those seeking to take their flexibility training to the next level, Proprioceptive Neuromuscular Facilitation (PNF) stretching offers a powerful and effective approach. PNF goes beyond traditional static stretches, utilizing reflexes and muscle contractions to achieve deeper stretches and improve flexibility. This section delves into the science behind PNF, explores various PNF techniques, and provides guidelines for safe and effective implementation.

Understanding PNF: The Science Behind the Stretch

PNF techniques target the body's neuromuscular system, specifically the muscle spindle and Golgi tendon organ (GTO) reflexes. Muscle spindles are sensory receptors within muscles that respond to stretch by sending signals to the nervous system to contract the muscle (stretch reflex). GTOs are located near tendons and respond to excessive tension by signaling the muscle to relax (inverse myotatic reflex). PNF techniques utilize these reflexes to achieve a deeper stretch than traditional static methods.

Types of PNF Stretches:

There are several PNF stretching techniques, each with slight variations. Here are three common methods:

- **Hold-Relax (Contract-Relax):**
  1. Stretch the target muscle to a point of mild tension (static hold for 10-15 seconds).
  2. Isometrically contract the stretched muscle against resistance for 7-15 seconds (e.g., pushing against a wall for a hamstring stretch).
  3. Relax the muscle completely.

4. Immediately re-stretch the target muscle. You should be able to achieve a deeper stretch due to the relaxed state of the muscle after the contraction.

- **Agonist Contract (Hold-Assist-Contract):**
    1. Stretch the target muscle to a point of mild tension (static hold for 10-15 seconds).
    2. Briefly contract the stretched muscle isometrically (without movement) for a few seconds.
    3. While holding the isometric contraction, a partner assists you in pushing the stretch slightly further.
    4. Relax the muscle completely.
    5. Re-stretch the target muscle. This technique utilizes the agonist muscle (the primary mover in a joint action) to facilitate a deeper stretch.
- **Contract-Relax with Agonist Contract (CRAC):** This combines elements of the

Hold-Relax and Agonist Contract techniques. It involves a static hold, isometric contraction, partner-assisted stretch, relaxation, and then another isometric contraction of the stretched muscle before the final re-stretch.

Benefits and Considerations for PNF Stretching:

Benefits:

- **Increased Flexibility:** PNF has been shown to be more effective than static stretching in achieving and maintaining greater flexibility gains.
- **Improved Muscle Strength:** The isometric contractions incorporated in PNF can also contribute to building strength in the stretched muscle.
- **Enhanced Neuromuscular Efficiency:** PNF can improve communication between the nervous system and muscles, leading to more coordinated movements.

Considerations:

- **Advanced Technique:** PNF requires proper technique and can be more challenging to perform than static stretches. Consider seeking guidance from a qualified professional to learn proper form.
- **Not for Everyone:** PNF is not suitable for everyone, especially those with certain injuries or medical conditions. Consult a healthcare professional before attempting PNF stretches.
- **Increased Intensity:** PNF stretches can be more intense than static stretches, so listen to your body and avoid pushing yourself to the point of pain.

Tips for Safe and Effective PNF Stretching:

- **Warm-up Properly:** Always perform a light cardio warm-up and dynamic stretches before attempting PNF techniques.

- **Focus on Form:** Proper form is crucial to maximize benefits and minimize the risk of injury. Consider working with a qualified professional to learn proper PNF techniques.
- **Breathe Deeply:** Maintain slow, deep breaths throughout the hold, contraction, and relaxation phases of the stretch.
- **Listen to Your Body:** Pain is a sign to stop. If you experience any pain during a PNF stretch, stop immediately and consult a healthcare professional.
- **Start Slowly:** Begin with shorter durations (hold times and contractions) and gradually increase them as your flexibility improves.

PNF stretching can be a powerful tool for athletes and fitness enthusiasts seeking to maximize their flexibility and performance. However, it's important to approach PNF cautiously, with proper technique and guidance, to ensure a safe and effective experience.

Remember: Consistency is key! Regularly incorporating PNF techniques into your stretching routine, along with other flexibility exercises, can lead to significant improvements in your range of motion and overall well-being.

Unveiling the Power of PNF Stretching: A Deep Dive into Techniques and Benefits

Proprioceptive Neuromuscular Facilitation (PNF) stretching offers a unique and effective approach to improve flexibility and performance. Unlike traditional static stretches, PNF techniques delve deeper, utilizing the body's neuromuscular system to achieve significant gains in range of motion. This comprehensive guide explores the science behind PNF, delves into various techniques, and provides insights for safe and effective implementation.

The Science of PNF Stretching:

PNF techniques target the body's intricate network of nerves and muscles, specifically the muscle spindle and Golgi tendon organ (GTO) reflexes. Muscle spindles act as sensory receptors within muscles. When stretched, they send signals to the nervous system to contract the muscle (stretch reflex). GTOs, located near tendons, respond to excessive tension by signaling the muscle to relax (inverse myotatic reflex). PNF techniques strategically utilize these reflexes to achieve deeper stretches than traditional static methods.

Popular PNF Techniques:

There are several PNF stretching techniques, each offering slight variations. Here's a breakdown of three common methods:

- **Hold-Relax (Contract-Relax):**
    1. **Static Hold (10-15 seconds):** Stretch the target muscle to a point of mild tension and hold for 10-15 seconds.
    2. **Isometric Contraction (7-15 seconds):** Contract the stretched muscle isometrically against resistance for 7-15 seconds (e.g., pushing against a wall for a hamstring stretch).
    3. **Relaxation:** Completely relax the muscle.

4. **Re-Stretch:** Immediately re-stretch the target muscle. Due to the relaxed state of the muscle after the contraction, you should be able to achieve a deeper stretch.

- **Agonist Contract (Hold-Assist-Contract):**
    1. **Static Hold (10-15 seconds):** Stretch the target muscle to a point of mild tension and hold for 10-15 seconds.
    2. **Isometric Contraction (few seconds):** Briefly contract the stretched muscle isometrically (without movement) for a few seconds.
    3. **Partner-Assisted Stretch:** While holding the isometric contraction, a partner assists you in pushing the stretch slightly further.
    4. **Relaxation:** Relax the muscle completely.
    5. **Re-Stretch:** Re-stretch the target muscle. This technique utilizes the

agonist muscle (the primary mover in a joint action) to facilitate a deeper stretch.

- **Contract-Relax with Agonist Contract (CRAC):**
- This combines elements of both Hold-Relax and Agonist Contract techniques. It involves a static hold, isometric contraction, partner-assisted stretch, relaxation, and then another isometric contraction of the stretched muscle before the final re-stretch.

Benefits of PNF Stretching:

The unique approach of PNF offers several advantages over traditional stretching methods:

- **Enhanced Flexibility:** Studies have shown PNF to be more effective than static stretches in achieving and maintaining greater flexibility gains.
- **Improved Muscle Strength:** The isometric contractions incorporated in

PNF can also contribute to building strength in the stretched muscle.

- **Enhanced Neuromuscular Efficiency:** PNF helps improve communication between the nervous system and muscles, leading to more coordinated movements.
- **Specificity:** PNF techniques can be tailored to target specific muscle groups, making them highly effective for athletes seeking to improve performance in their sport.

Considerations and Safety Tips:

While PNF offers significant benefits, there are crucial aspects to consider for safe and effective implementation:

- **Advanced Technique:** PNF requires proper technique and can be more challenging to perform than static stretches. Consider seeking guidance from a certified healthcare professional or physical therapist to learn proper form.

- **Not for Everyone:** PNF is not suitable for everyone, particularly those with certain injuries or medical conditions. Consult a healthcare professional before attempting PNF stretches.
- **Increased Intensity:** PNF stretches can be more intense than static stretches. Focus on proper form, listen to your body, and avoid pushing yourself to the point of pain.

Optimizing Your PNF Stretching Experience:

Here are some tips to ensure a safe and effective PNF stretching routine:

- **Warm-up Properly:** Always perform a light cardio warm-up and dynamic stretches before attempting PNF techniques.
- **Focus on Form:** Proper form is crucial to maximize benefits and minimize the risk of injury. Consider working with a qualified professional to learn proper PNF techniques.

- **Breathe Deeply:** Maintain slow, deep breaths throughout the hold, contraction, and relaxation phases of the stretch.
- **Listen to Your Body:** Pain is a sign to stop. If you experience any pain during a PNF stretch, stop immediately and consult a healthcare professional.

Chapter 11

Safety Considerations and Modifications for Stretching

Stretching is a fantastic way to improve flexibility, reduce muscle tension, and enhance overall well-being. However, it's crucial to prioritize safety throughout your stretching routine. Here's a breakdown of key safety considerations, how to differentiate between discomfort and pain, and some modifications to make stretching accessible for everyone.

Safety First:

- **Warm Up:** Always perform a light cardio warm-up (5-10 minutes) and dynamic stretches before static stretching. This prepares your muscles for movement and reduces the risk of injury.
- **Listen to Your Body:** Pay attention to your body's signals. Stretching should feel like a gentle pulling sensation, not sharp

pain. If you experience pain, stop the stretch immediately.

- **Maintain Proper Form:** Don't bounce or force stretches. Aim for smooth, controlled movements and proper alignment. Consider consulting a healthcare professional or fitness instructor to learn proper form for specific stretches.
- **Hold for Appropriate Durations:** Generally, hold static stretches for 15-30 seconds each. Avoid holding your breath while stretching.
- **Breathe Deeply:** Focus on slow, deep breaths throughout your stretches. Inhale through your nose and exhale slowly through your mouth.

Knowing When to Stop: Discomfort vs. Pain

The line between discomfort and pain can be subtle. Here's a helpful guide:

- **Discomfort:** This is a normal sensation during stretching, especially when targeting tight muscles. It feels like a gentle pulling or tension and usually subsides as you hold the stretch.

- **Pain:** This is a sharp, burning sensation and a signal to stop the stretch immediately. Pain indicates potential injury and should not be ignored.

Stretching Modifications for Everyone:

Stretching should be accessible for everyone, regardless of age, fitness level, or limitations. Here are some modifications to make stretches more inclusive:

- **Use Props:** Straps, yoga blocks, or towels can be used to deepen or modify stretches to make them more accessible.
- **Reduce Range of Motion:** Don't force yourself to go beyond your comfortable range of motion. Gradually increase the intensity of your stretches over time.
- **Chair Stretches:** Many stretches can be adapted to be done while seated in a chair,

making them suitable for those with limited mobility.

- **Focus on Breath:** Focus on your breath and relaxation throughout the stretches. This can help reduce tension and improve the overall experience.

Sample Stretching Exercises (considering modifications):

Upper Body:

- **Neck Stretch (Modified):** Sit or stand tall and slowly tilt your head to one side, bringing your ear towards your shoulder. Hold for 15-30 seconds and repeat on the other side (consider using a hand to guide your head gently, not forcing the stretch).
- **Arm Circles (Slow and Controlled):** Stand tall with your arms outstretched to the sides at shoulder height. Make slow, controlled circles forward and backward for 10 repetitions each direction (can be done seated in a chair).

- **Doorway Chest Opener (Modified):** Stand in a doorway with your forearms on either side of the frame at a lower level (approximately chest height). Gently lean forward, feeling a mild stretch across your chest and shoulders. Hold for 15-30 seconds (consider reducing the depth of the stretch if needed).

Lower Body:

- **Hamstring Stretch (Supine with Strap):** Lie on your back with both legs extended. Loop a yoga strap or towel around the arch of one foot and gently pull it towards you, feeling a stretch in the back of your thigh. Hold for 15-30 seconds and repeat on the other side (the strap can be used to assist you in reaching your foot comfortably).
- **Quad Stretch (Modified):** Lie on your stomach or stand with one leg bent behind you, grasping your ankle (whichever position feels more comfortable). Gently

squeeze your glutes of the bent leg. Hold for 15-30 seconds and repeat on the other side (consider using a strap or towel to assist you in reaching your ankle if needed).

Remember: Stretching is a journey, not a destination. Be patient, listen to your body, and gradually increase the intensity and duration of your stretches over time. With consistency and proper form, you'll reap the numerous benefits of stretching and move with greater ease and flexibility.

Stretching with Injuries or Medical Conditions: Safety First

Stretching offers a multitude of benefits, but it's crucial to approach it with caution if you have any injuries or medical conditions. Certain stretches may exacerbate existing issues, so consulting a healthcare professional before embarking on a stretching routine is vital. Here's a breakdown of key considerations for safe stretching with injuries or medical conditions.

Why Consulting a Healthcare Professional Matters:

- **Understanding Your Limitations:** A healthcare professional can assess your specific injury or condition and recommend safe and effective stretches that won't worsen your situation.
- **Modified Stretches:** They can provide modifications for existing stretches or suggest alternative stretches that target the same muscle groups while avoiding potential aggravation.

- **Guidance on Healing:** They can guide you on incorporating stretches into your recovery plan to promote healing and improve flexibility once your injury starts to mend.

General Considerations for Stretching with Injuries:

- **Focus on Pain Management:** Pain is a red flag. If a stretch causes any pain, stop immediately and consult your healthcare professional.
- **Prioritize Gentle Stretches:** Opt for gentle stretches that target the surrounding muscles rather than directly stressing the injured area.
- **Reduced Range of Motion:** Don't push yourself beyond your comfortable range of motion. Focus on controlled movements and gradual improvement.
- **Listen to Your Body:** Pay close attention to how your body feels during and after stretches. Any lingering pain or

discomfort is a sign to modify or stop the stretch.

- **Focus on Breath:** Deep, diaphragmatic breathing can help promote relaxation and reduce tension throughout your stretches.

Additional Tips:

- **Heat Therapy:** Applying heat (warm compress or light shower) before stretching can help loosen tight muscles and prepare them for movement. However, always consult your healthcare professional before using heat therapy, especially if you have certain medical conditions.
- **Ice Therapy:** After stretching, ice therapy (ice pack wrapped in a towel) can help reduce inflammation and promote healing, especially for acute injuries. Again, consult your healthcare professional before using ice therapy.
- **Maintain a Healthy Lifestyle:** Getting enough sleep, eating a balanced diet, and staying hydrated can all contribute to the

healing process and support your body's recovery.

Remember: When in doubt, leave it out. It's always better to err on the side of caution and prioritize your safety. A healthcare professional can be your best resource for creating a safe and effective stretching routine that complements your healing journey.

Chapter 12

The Lifelong Benefits of Flexibility

Embracing Mobility and Independence: A Guide for Active Aging

As we age, the thought of maintaining mobility and independence can become a growing concern. However, with a proactive approach, you can empower yourself to stay active, manage limitations, and live a fulfilling life on your own terms. This guide explores various strategies to promote mobility, preserve independence, and embrace the joys of active aging.

The Importance of Mobility and Independence:

- **Quality of Life:** Maintaining mobility allows you to engage in daily activities, pursue hobbies, and participate in social interactions, all of which contribute to a richer quality of life.

- **Physical and Mental Well-being:** Regular physical activity can improve cardiovascular health, strengthen bones and muscles, and boost cognitive function.
- **Reduced Reliance on Others:** Maintaining independence allows you to manage your daily tasks without needing constant assistance, fostering a sense of self-sufficiency and dignity.

Strategies for Maintaining Mobility:

- **Exercise Regularly:** Aim for at least 30 minutes of moderate-intensity exercise most days of the week. This can include walking, swimming, cycling, dancing, or low-impact aerobics.
- **Strength Training:** Incorporate strength training exercises at least twice a week to maintain muscle mass and bone density. Bodyweight exercises, resistance bands, or light weights can be effective tools.

- **Balance and Flexibility Exercises:** Regularly practice balance exercises like heel-toe walking or tai chi to improve stability and reduce the risk of falls. Stretching exercises can help maintain flexibility and improve range of motion.
- **Physical Therapy:** Consulting a physical therapist can be highly beneficial. They can develop a personalized exercise program to address specific limitations and improve overall mobility.

Enhancing Independence in Daily Living:

- **Home Modifications:** Consider making modifications to your home to enhance safety and accessibility. This may include installing grab bars in bathrooms, adding ramps to doorways, or using raised toilet seats.
- **Assistive Devices:** Explore assistive devices like canes, walkers, or grabber tools to help you perform daily tasks safely and independently.

- **Smart Home Technology:** Smart home features like voice-activated lighting or thermostats can simplify daily tasks and promote independence.
- **Meal Planning and Preparation:** Plan and prepare healthy meals in advance to ensure you have nutritious options readily available. Consider online grocery delivery services or meal kit subscriptions for added convenience.
- **Transportation Options:** If driving becomes a challenge, explore alternative transportation options like public transportation, ride-sharing services, or senior transportation programs.

Additional Tips for Active Aging:

- **Maintain a Healthy Diet:** Eating a balanced diet rich in fruits, vegetables, whole grains, and lean protein ensures your body receives the nutrients it needs to function optimally.
- **Stay Hydrated:** Drinking plenty of water throughout the day is crucial for overall

health and can help prevent dehydration, which can impact mobility and cognitive function.

- **Socialize Regularly:** Social interaction helps combat loneliness and isolation, which can contribute to a decline in well-being. Stay connected with friends and family, join social groups, or volunteer in your community.
- **Regular Checkups:** Schedule regular checkups with your doctor to monitor your health and address any potential concerns early on.
- **Mental Stimulation:** Engage in activities that stimulate your mind, such as reading, playing games, or learning a new skill.

Embracing an Active Lifestyle:

Maintaining mobility and independence as we age is not just about limitations; it's about embracing an active and fulfilling lifestyle. By incorporating these strategies into your routine, you can empower yourself to stay active, manage challenges, and continue living life to the fullest. Remember, you are not alone on this journey. There are numerous resources available to support you, from healthcare professionals and physical therapists to community programs and senior centers. Take charge of your well-being, embrace the possibilities of active aging, and continue living a life filled with mobility, independence, and joy.

Stretch Your Way to a Healthier, Happier You: A Guide to Stretching for All

Stretching is often an overlooked yet powerful tool for promoting a healthy and active lifestyle. It offers a wide range of benefits, from improved flexibility and injury prevention to better sleep and stress reduction. This comprehensive guide explores the world of stretching, providing you with the knowledge and practical tips to integrate stretching seamlessly into your daily routine.

Unlocking the Benefits of Stretching:

- **Enhanced Flexibility:** Regular stretching helps lengthen and loosen your muscles, allowing for a wider range of motion in your joints. This translates to smoother movement in daily activities and potentially improved performance in your favorite sports.
- **Reduced Injury Risk:** Tight muscles are more prone to tears and strains. Stretching helps maintain muscle elasticity, allowing

them to absorb force and adapt to sudden movements, thus reducing the likelihood of injuries.

- **Improved Posture:** Stretching can help counteract the postural imbalances caused by prolonged sitting or repetitive motions. By targeting tight muscles and strengthening opposing muscle groups, you can achieve better posture, leading to less pain and discomfort.
- **Stress Reduction and Relaxation:** Stretching encourages mindfulness and focuses your attention on your breath and body sensations. This can help quiet a racing mind and promote a sense of calm, especially when incorporated into a pre-bed routine.
- **Enhanced Circulation:** Gentle stretching can improve blood flow throughout your body, promoting relaxation and aiding in the removal of metabolic waste products that can contribute to fatigue.

Crafting Your Stretching Routine:

Here are some key considerations to create a personalized stretching routine:

- **Target Different Muscle Groups:** Aim to stretch all major muscle groups in your body, including your upper body (neck, shoulders, back), core, and lower body (hamstrings, quadriceps, calves).
- **Hold Stretches for Appropriate Durations:** Generally, hold static stretches for 15-30 seconds each. Avoid bouncing or forcing stretches. Aim for a gentle pulling sensation.
- **Listen to Your Body:** Pain is a sign to stop the stretch immediately. Stretching should feel good, not cause discomfort.
- **Breathe Deeply:** Focus on slow, deep breaths throughout your stretches. Inhale through your nose and exhale slowly through your mouth.
- **Consider the Timing:** Stretching can be done at various times throughout the day. Here are some suggestions:

- **Morning Stretches:** Wake up your muscles and improve circulation with some gentle stretches before your day begins.
- **Post-Workout Stretches:** Dedicate 5-10 minutes after a workout to focus on stretches that target areas like your lower back, shoulders, and hamstrings.
- **Pre-Bed Stretches:** Wind down before bed with some relaxing stretches to ease muscle tension and promote better sleep.

Simple Stretches for Everyday Integration:

Here are some basic stretches you can easily incorporate into your routine:

- **Neck Stretch:** Sit or stand tall and slowly tilt your head to one side, bringing your ear towards your shoulder. Hold for 15-30 seconds and repeat on the other side.
- **Shoulder Roll:** Lift your shoulders up towards your ears, roll them back and

down in a circular motion. Repeat 5-10 times in each direction.

- **Hamstring Stretch:** Lie on your back with one leg extended. Loop a yoga strap or towel around the arch of your foot and gently pull it towards you. Hold for 15-30 seconds and repeat on the other side.
- **Quad Stretch:** Stand on one leg, holding onto a chair or wall for balance. Gently pull your other foot up behind you, grabbing your ankle or calf muscle. Hold for 15-30 seconds and repeat on the other side.

Beyond the Basics: Exploring Different Stretching Techniques:

As you progress, consider exploring different stretching techniques for a more comprehensive approach:

- **Static Stretching:** Holding a stretch in a fixed position for a specific duration.
- **Dynamic Stretching:** Active movements that prepare your muscles for activity.

- **PNF Stretching (Proprioceptive Neuromuscular Facilitation):** A more advanced technique that utilizes reflexes to achieve deeper stretches (consult a healthcare professional before attempting PNF).

Remember: Consistency is key! Make stretching a regular habit, and you'll be well on your way to reaping the numerous benefits it offers. Stretch often, move with ease, and feel the difference in your overall well-being!

Glossary

This glossary provides definitions for commonly encountered terms used in the world of stretching:

- **Agonist Muscle:** The primary muscle responsible for movement in a joint action (e.g., the quadriceps muscle is the agonist in a knee extension).
- **Antagonist Muscle:** The muscle that opposes the action of the agonist muscle (e.g., the hamstrings are the antagonists to the quadriceps in a knee extension).
- **Ballistic Stretching:** A bouncing type of stretch where momentum is used to force the body beyond its normal range of motion (generally not recommended due to increased risk of injury).
- **Dynamic Stretching:** Active movements that prepare the muscles for activity and improve range of motion (e.g., leg swings, arm circles).

- **Flexibility:** The range of motion in a joint or group of joints.
- **Hold-Relax (Contract-Relax):** A PNF stretching technique where a static stretch is held, followed by an isometric contraction, relaxation, and then a re-stretch.
- **Isometric Contraction:** A muscle contraction where the muscle length remains the same, but tension increases (e.g., pushing against a wall during a hamstring stretch).
- **Myofascial Release:** A technique using self-massage tools or sustained pressure to target tightness and trigger points in the fascia (connective tissue) and muscles.
- **Muscle Spindle:** A sensory receptor within a muscle that responds to stretch by sending signals to the nervous system to contract the muscle (stretch reflex).
- **Passive Stretching:** A stretch where an external force (e.g., partner assistance, yoga strap) is used to achieve a deeper stretch.

- **PNF Stretching (Proprioceptive Neuromuscular Facilitation):** An advanced stretching technique that utilizes reflexes to achieve deeper stretches.
- **Range of Motion (ROM):** The extent of movement possible in a joint.
- **Static Stretching:** Holding a stretch in a fixed position for a specific duration (15-30 seconds is common).
- **Trigger Point:** A hypersensitive area within a muscle that can cause pain and referred pain in other parts of the body.

Additional Terms:

- **Active Stretching:** Stretching a muscle by actively contracting it in opposition to the one you're stretching (e.g., quad stretch with hip flexor contraction).
- **Hold-Assist-Contract (Agonist Contract):** A PNF stretching technique involving a static hold, partner-assisted stretch, and an isometric contraction of the stretched muscle.

- **Golgi Tendon Organ (GTO):** A sensory receptor located near a tendon that responds to excessive tension by signaling the muscle to relax (inverse myotatic reflex).

I hope this glossary helps you navigate the world of stretching terminology!

Other Material

Sample Stretching Routines Tailored for Your Needs:

Here are a few example stretching routines designed to target specific needs and fitness levels:

Gentle Morning Stretches (5-10 minutes):

- Focus: Waking up your body and improving circulation.
- Suitable for: All fitness levels.
- Cat-Cow Stretch: Begin on all fours with hands shoulder-width apart and knees hip-width apart. As you inhale, arch your back and lift your head (cow pose). As you exhale, round your back and tuck your chin (cat pose). Repeat 5-10 times.
- Supine Arm Circles: Lie on your back with arms outstretched to the sides at shoulder height. Make slow, controlled circles forward and backward for 10 repetitions each direction.

- Neck Stretch (Modified): Sit or stand tall and slowly tilt your head to one side, bringing your ear towards your shoulder. Hold for 15-30 seconds and repeat on the other side (consider using a hand to guide your head gently, not forcing the stretch).
- Seated Hamstring Stretch: Sit on the floor with both legs extended. Gently reach for your toes, keeping your back straight (use a yoga strap if needed). Hold for 15-30 seconds.

Post-Workout Cool Down (10-15 minutes):

- Focus: Targeting major muscle groups used during your workout and improving flexibility.
- Suitable for: All fitness levels, with modifications for higher-intensity workouts.
- Quad Stretch: Stand on one leg, holding onto a chair or wall for balance. Gently pull your other foot up behind you, grabbing your ankle or calf muscle. Hold

for 15-30 seconds and repeat on the other side (consider modifying for high-impact workouts by using a wall or strap for deeper stretch).

- Chest Opener (Doorway): Stand in a doorway with your forearms on either side of the frame at a lower level (approximately chest height). Gently lean forward, feeling a mild stretch across your chest and shoulders. Hold for 15-30 seconds.
- Calf Raises: Stand with your feet shoulder-width apart and slowly rise up onto your toes. Hold for a few seconds, then lower your heels back down. Repeat 10-15 times.
- Lower Back Rotation: Lie on your back with knees bent and feet flat on the floor. Slowly turn your knees to one side, keeping your shoulders flat on the ground. Hold for 15-30 seconds, then repeat on the other side.

Pre-Bed Relaxation Stretches (5-10 minutes):

- Focus: Winding down for better sleep and reducing muscle tension.
- Suitable for: All fitness levels.
- Happy Baby Pose: Lie on your back with knees bent and feet flat on the floor. Bring your knees towards your chest and grasp the outside of your feet with your hands. Gently rock back and forth for a few minutes.
- Supine Twist: Lie on your back with arms outstretched to the sides. Slowly lower both knees to one side, keeping your shoulders flat on the ground. Hold for 15-30 seconds, then repeat on the other side.
- Seated Piriformis Stretch: Sit on the floor with one leg crossed over the other knee. Gently lean forward from your hips, feeling a stretch in your glutes. Hold for 15-30 scconds and repeat on the other side.
- Deep Breaths: Focus on slow, deep breaths throughout your stretches. Inhale

through your nose and exhale slowly through your mouth.

Remember: These are just examples. You can customize them based on your individual needs and preferences. Listen to your body, don't bounce, and hold stretches for a comfortable duration.

Additional Tips:

- Warm up before stretching with light cardio or dynamic stretches (especially before a post-workout routine).
- Breathe deeply and slowly throughout your stretches.
- Focus on proper form over intensity.
- If you experience any pain, stop the stretch immediately.
- Consult a healthcare professional before starting any new stretching routine, especially if you have any injuries or medical conditions.

With these sample routines and a little exploration, you can find a stretching practice that perfectly complements your lifestyle and helps you move with more ease and flexibility. Happy stretching!

Stretch: Neck Stretch (Modified)

Description:

- Sit or stand tall with your shoulders relaxed and back straight.
- Gently tilt your head to one side, bringing your ear towards your shoulder.
- Maintain a neutral gaze (don't look up or down).
- You should feel a mild stretch along the side of your neck and upper shoulder.

Instructions:

1. Find a comfortable seated or standing position. Maintain good posture with your shoulders relaxed and back straight.

2. Slowly begin to tilt your head to one side, bringing your ear closer to your shoulder. Imagine your ear is trying to gently touch your shoulder.
3. Keep your chin slightly tucked in and avoid looking up or down. Focus on lengthening the side of your neck.
4. Hold this position for 15-30 seconds, breathing deeply and slowly throughout.
5. Gently return to the starting position and repeat the stretch on the other side.

Additional Tips:

- If you don't feel a stretch, try tilting your head slightly forward.
- Avoid forcing the stretch or using any jerky movements.
- If you experience any pain, stop the stretch immediately.

Alternative:

For those with limited neck mobility, consider a modified version:

- Sit or stand tall and maintain good posture.
- Gently place one hand on the top of your head, palm facing down.
- Apply gentle downward pressure on your head, guiding it slightly towards your shoulder. Avoid pushing too hard.
- Hold for 15-30 seconds, breathing deeply.
- Repeat on the other side.

By following these descriptions and instructions, you can perform a safe and effective neck stretch. This approach can be applied to other stretches, providing clear guidance without potentially unsafe visuals.

Request for reviews

Hi everyone!

I'm so excited to finally announce that my book, *"Stretching for a Healthy and Active Lifestyle"*, is now available!

This book has been a labor of love, pouring all my knowledge and passion for stretching into a resource that can empower people of all ages and abilities to move with more ease and enjoy the benefits of flexibility.

Whether you're a seasoned athlete looking to optimize your performance or someone simply wanting to stay active and manage everyday aches and pains, I believe this book has something to offer you.

Here's what you can expect:

- **Simple and Effective Stretches:** Easy-to-follow instructions with clear explanations to guide you through safe and beneficial stretches.

- **Personalized Routines:** Tailored approaches for different needs and fitness levels, helping you create a stretching routine that fits your lifestyle.
- **Benefits Beyond Flexibility:** Explore the positive impact stretching can have on your overall well-being, from stress reduction to improved sleep.

If you've had a chance to check out the book, I'd be incredibly grateful if you could leave a review .

Your honest feedback is invaluable, not only for me as an author, but also for helping others discover the potential of stretching in their lives.

Happy stretching!

Warmly,

Helen Talbott

https://go.screenpal.com/watch/cZev2xVscR8
Video link for tutorials

www.ingramcontent.com/pod-product-compliance
Lightning Source LLC
Chambersburg PA
CBHW081211260726
48653CB00010BA/3600